PAINFUL

PAINFUL SEX

A guide to causes, treatments and prevention

Michele Goldsmith

Thorsons
An Imprint of HarperCollins*Publishers*

Thorsons
An Imprint of HarperCollins*Publishers*
77–85 Fulham Palace Road,
Hammersmith, London W6 8JB
1160 Battery Street,
San Francisco, California 94111–1213

Published by Thorsons 1995

3 5 7 9 10 8 6 4 2 1

© Michele Goldsmith 1995

Michele Goldsmith asserts the moral right to
be identified as the author of this work

Text illustrations by Peter Cox

A catalogue record for this book
is available from the British Library

ISBN 0 7225 3104 4

Printed in Great Britain by
HarperCollinsManufacturing Glasgow

All rights reserved. No part of this publication may be
reproduced, stored in a retrieval system, or transmitted,
in any form or by any means, electronic, mechanical,
photocopying, storage or otherwise, without the prior
permission of the publishers.

Contents

Acknowledgements vii
Introduction ix

1 Vaginal Infections and Irritations 1
2 Non-infectious Causes of Vaginal Pain 32
3 Causes of Deep Internal Pain 63
4 The Emotional Effects of Painful Sex 85
5 Infertility 104
6 Choosing a Complementary Therapy 111

Bibliography 118
Useful Addresses 121
Index 133

Acknowledgements

I dedicate this book to Dr George Atallah and all the women at the vestibulitis support group with the hope that we may find an effective cure for this distressing condition. Thanks also to my partner Anthony Harris for his selfless love and emotional support, my cousin Julie Winkler and my brother Simon Goldsmith for their assistance, and all the women who shared their experiences with me to make this book possible.

I would also like to thank Dr J. White, Genito Urinary Physician at the Department of Sexual Medicine at Heartlands Hospital, Birmingham, England; Dr George Morrison at the Genito Urinary Department at the Freedom Fields Hospital, Plymouth; Penny Sargent and Carol Sutton at Plymouth University, England; Dr John Studd, Gynaecologist at King's College Hospital, Denmark Hill, London, England; Dr Angela Robinson, Mortimer Market Clinic, London, England and Dr Heather Montford, Psychosexual Counsellor at the Margaret Pyke Centre, London, England for providing information.

INTRODUCTION

I am 28 years old and have been sexually active for the last nine years, but I have almost always associated sex with pain – a bewildering pain with a variety of names which I never really understood. I grew up a 'liberated', fun-loving woman, fully in tune with my sexuality and fully expecting to be able to express it like any other young adult, yet very often I could not. This book springs from the distress and isolation I felt when sex itself became a difficulty for me.

I first went to a gynaecologist about painful sex when I was 19. He told me that changing positions might make things easier, which it did for a while. During my early twenties, I often had to take large doses of antibiotics for recurring tonsillitis which in turn gave me the disastrous cyclical problems of persistent cystitis and thrush (yeast infection). It seemed that while my contemporaries were enjoying hassle-free, healthy sex lives, I was being systematically 'punished' for such things and this made my discovery of sexual pleasure thoroughly miserable. It made me angry that the incidence and frequency of these two conditions, which affect thousands of women physically, sexually and emotionally, seemed to be taken as routine by doctors. Indeed, their endemic occurrence was often offered as a bizarre panacea to my suffering. Comments such as 'lots of women get recurrent thrush (yeast infection), it is really common', do not really help when you are faced with an angry, frustrated partner and another uncomfortable day sitting at your desk.

The causes of these conditions were never investigated, I was rarely examined thoroughly and the treatment offered seemed to be very limited. From these experiences, I quickly learned that painful sex, like painful periods, is something many women are expected to just grin and bear because nobody is really very interested.

After a brief reprieve in my mid-twenties, I experienced another bout of symptoms similar to thrush (yeast infection), yet none of the usual treatments seemed to clear it up. My symptoms were so severe that sometimes the pain kept me up all night and I could not have any sexual contact because my genital area was so tender and painful. I was completely panic-stricken and convinced that there was something terribly wrong with me. Having had no luck with my GP, I visited a genito-urinary clinic, formerly known as a sexually transmitted diseases (STD) clinic. After many painful tests the doctors there said they could not find anything wrong and gave me a cream to soothe this 'phantom' itching. This convinced me that perhaps I had developed a psychological aversion to sex. After a further six months of suffering I was referred once again to a gynaecologist. After a short examination he knew immediately what was wrong. I remember hearing him gently explain, 'You are not imagining it. You have a condition known as vulval vestibulitis. Now get dressed and I will tell you what we can do about it.'

Although the name itself meant nothing, I instantly burst into tears – tears of relief mixed with furious anger. Why had it not been diagnosed before? How many other women think this pain is all in their heads? After some research, I discovered that vulval vestibulitis had been written about and discussed in numerous medical journals since 1980 – this was 1991.

As a result of my own experiences and the letters I have received from other women after sharing my story in women's magazines, I have been inspired to write a guide for women who find sex painful and want to understand why and what can be done about it. Dyspareunia is the medical term and covers many conditions that can give rise to painful sex. Hopefully, this book will help create awareness of these conditions so that they get the attention they deserve.

When Sex Goes Wrong

Since the introduction of free contraception and the birth control pill in the 1960s, women have had more control and choice regarding their sexual relations. This control means that today, having an enjoyable, healthy sex life is easily taken for granted and, that for most of us, it is a natural, desirable and spontaneous part of life. Given this background, I was amazed to discover that a huge number of women find sex painful. An American survey by Aaron Glatt, which attempted to quantify the incidence of painful sex, discovered that over 60 per cent of women have had problems with painful sex at some point in their lives[1]. Glatt's survey looked specifically at the incidence of painful penetrative intercourse, so unfortunately we do not know the statistics concerning other sexual practices. He concentrated on a group of heterosexual women in their early thirties who had been sexually active for between 10 and 20 years. Of the women who suffered from painful sex, it was found that a third had pain only during initial penetration, a third had pain throughout intercourse and a third had pain only after intercourse. To a great extent the women were alone in their suffering. Most had discussed the problem with their partners, but very few had consulted a close friend or relative. Less surprising is that many of the women had noticed an adverse affect on their relationships. Perhaps most disturbing of all is that most of the women did not consult a doctor or health care professional about their pain. Of those of who did, *only a third received a specific diagnosis and treatment.*

I want to qualify here that I do not believe that women need to be able to have penetrative sex to have a complete and loving sex life and no woman should ever be made to feel abnormal about her sexual preferences. However, I think everybody has a right to a choice. Very often painful sex can mean that any gentle pressure around the vaginal area, not just intercourse, is painful. This is not normal and every woman has the right to be taken seriously and the problem to be investigated properly.

The Cost

When sex is not simple and straightforward, it can easily change from being a joyous experience into a source of physical and emotional distress. This distress is severely exacerbated if the cause of the pain cannot be found and a woman feels she has no one to turn to. There are many emotional reasons why sex can be a painful experience for some women, including a history of sexual abuse or a traumatic incident such as rape. Unfortunately these issues will not be dealt with here as they are outside the remit of this book, and deserve examination on their own.

But whatever the reasons, feeling unable to have a trouble-free sexual relationship, especially with someone you love, is like being banished to the fringes of a world that has deliberately excluded you. When my vestibulitis forced me to abstain from intercourse with my long-term boyfriend for almost a year, there were times when I could not bear to watch the carefree, celebratory sex scenes of romantic films, or even to see couples caressing each other in the park. Many women who have had their sexual relationships disrupted for physical or psychological reasons have experienced similar feelings of freakishness, of not being a 'whole' woman and some women feel as if they are carrying an invisible disability. As we can see from some of the following experiences, painful sex can have a lasting effect on a woman's self-image, sexuality and fertility.

Am I Going Mad?

Sex has always been a horror for me and to some extent it still is. At first I thought it was meant to be like that, then I thought it was something to do with my periods, or the position I was having sex in. As soon as I began to feel aroused my abdomen would bloat out and become rock-hard. Intercourse felt as if someone had put a brick inside me and everything was being crushed. My boyfriend and I rarely continued beyond this point. When I was finally referred by my GP to the hospital, they diagnosed pelvic inflammatory disease (PID).

JANE, 23

At the birth of my first child I had an episiotomy which meant that the cut made around the vaginal entrance during labour had to be stitched up. I felt very sore for a long time afterwards and sex was impossible. After six months my doctor was still telling me it needed more time to heal and would get better on its own. It wasn't until I broke down in hysterical tears and demanded something should be done that I was referred to hospital for a simple operation that cured it. I couldn't help thinking that according to the doctor, I wasn't supposed to be sexual after I had a child.

SARAH, 30

When I was 23 I developed a soreness around my vagina that wouldn't go away. The specialists I went to see did lots of tests but didn't know what it was. The area was very red and swollen and

PAINFUL SEX

I couldn't bear to be touched, it was so painful. I carried around a whole bag of creams to try and soothe myself but nothing worked and I became allergic and immune to them. It was a very isolating experience; I was miserable all the time and I couldn't tell people why. It's only since I've been cured that I see how much vesitublitis changed my personality.

RUTH, 36

My recurrent thrush (yeast infection) makes me feel very dirty and unsexual. Sometimes I think I will never be normal down there again and every time I go to the doctor I seem to get the brush-off. If I see myself as dirty and undesirable, how can I expect my partner to see me as sexual? Many doctors also tell me that my partner should use treatments to avoid passing it between us, but this always causes conflict, and seems to do more harm than good.

LUCY, 26

As we can see, communicating difficulties in this area can be very awkward and one demoralizing rebuff from an unsympathetic or ill-informed doctor can sentence a woman to months or even years of further misery. As one woman wrote to me, 'the *pain* of painful sex is not being emotionally understood'.

Painful sex can be a way for our bodies to let us know that something is wrong; it could be an infection that will worsen and even affect fertility if left untreated. So it is important for women to learn to recognize these warning symptoms and feel comfortable about seeking medical advice for the sake of their general health. To do this we need to feel that doctors are *listening* to what we are telling them about our bodies. Very often the physical causes of painful sex seem to be too easily missed by doctors unless the symptoms are immediately obvious and detectable. When they are not at all obvious, many women are unnecessarily classified as having psychological problems. This dismissal can lead to feelings of isolation and stigmatization, a state which can put a woman's health at risk. As a consultant gynaecologist at the Whittington Hospital, Mr Singer explains 'If a woman is experiencing persistent vulval or pelvic pain she must see a specialist so that potentially harmful conditions such as cancers can be ruled out.'

The conditions that cause painful sex are under-diagnosed and underestimated by the medical profession for a variety of reasons. Most of the conditions affect only women and currently 78 per cent of gynaecologists and 74 per cent of GPs are men It seems that an unfortunate by-product of this imbalance has been a lack of vigorous interest in women's health issues, and in some cases, a systematic dismissal of these conditions as unimportant. In an era of limited health resources these conditions have taken a back seat on the priority list, especially since none of the conditions is life-threatening. Even the least cynical observer of the medical establishment can see that conditions such as thrush (yeast infection) and cystitis are seen as mundane 'ailments' and there is very little glamour and prestige attached to finding a cure for such things. It is also my own personal observation that over the last decade, budgets for research into sexual health have, quite rightly, been energetically channelled into finding treatments for HIV, and unfortunately, research into other sexually transmitted diseases may not have received the attention it deserves. However, the incidence of HIV means that the defence mechanisms of the vagina are now at last being researched and there may be more hope for the future.

The double standard over female sexuality still exists – the same sexual behaviour that is part of making a man a healthy, fun-loving 'lad', may lead to a woman being labelled promiscuous, and unfortunately, some doctors still make the link between troubles in the vaginal area with 'promiscuous' behaviour. Consequently, a woman is seen to have brought the problem on herself and does not merit sympathy. Another widely held notion is that women are expected to bear pain. In the light of period pains, childbirth trauma and so on, complaints of pain from a woman are more likely to be ignored or dismissed as natural, part of being a woman. Older women, in particular, who find that the menopause alters their sex life, discover that many doctors dismiss their sexual needs.

> *It took all the courage in the world for me to go to my GP and tell him that my husband and I had found making love difficult for the past three years. He told me to stop dwelling on it, that lots of women find this and it is not unusual. His solution was 'if it hurts, don't do it' and that was it. I was shattered.*
>
> ANGELA, 58

Presenting any symptoms to a doctor that defy a textbook definition can baffle and consequently alienate the doctor who is struggling to find a diagnosis. Remember that doctors are taught to cure and when they can not find a cause, they may get frustrated and take it out on the patient by saying it is all in her head.

The information and suggestions that follow may be helpful if you have not yet been able to discover an adequate explanation or cure for your problems. It will help you to discover what the problem is, why it occurs, how it affects you and how it can be diagnosed, treated and managed. The more you know, the more likely you are to obtain a proper diagnosis and treatment plan from medical advisors. Or you may need some support to cope with an already diagnosed condition which has disrupted something as fundamental as your sexual identity and fulfilment. Whatever the reason, I hope this book will help you to avoid unnecessary suffering and put you back on the path to enjoying your sexuality to the full.

Chapter 1
VAGINAL INFECTIONS AND IRRITATIONS

In the Introduction we learned that many women who find sex painful may be reluctant to seek help for their condition, or are unable to find the right sort of help. There may be many reasons for this, but one explanation for why women feel this diffidence might be the way in which women are brought up to see their bodies. Men have a penis which lays outside their body, which makes it easier for them to touch and explore their genitals. It is also easier for men to see where and how things work. Female genitalia is hidden, shrouded in mystery, and as a result, women have not been encouraged to touch and explore themselves in the way men seem able to do quite naturally. If you feel something is going wrong 'down there', you are less likely to seek help and advice if you feel uncomfortable about the area in the first place. For this reason alone, it is important to understand what your genitals look like (*see fig. 1*).

Exploring Yourself

It is easy to examine your own *vulva* if you sit down on the bed, bend your knees, then spread your legs apart and hold a mirror in front of the area between your upper thighs. Knowing where everything is and how a healthy vulva should look will also help you identify problems that may come up later in the book.

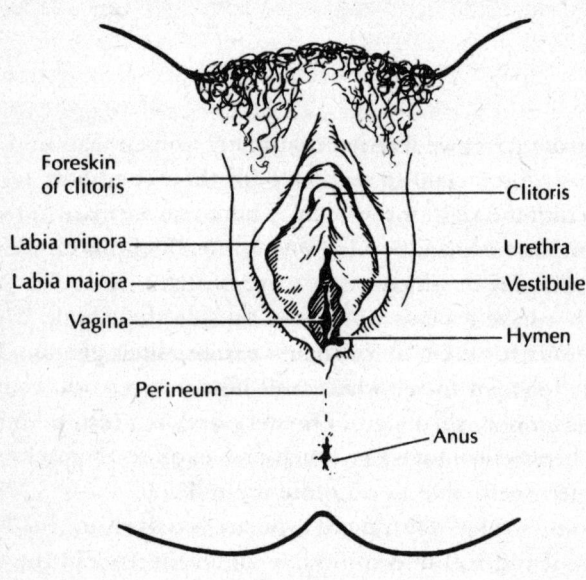

Figure 1

VAGINAL INFECTIONS AND IRRITATIONS

Just as your face has lips, so has the vulva; there are two sets which surround and protect the vaginal opening. The external lips, covered with pubic hair, are called the *labia majora*. These are two protective fatty cushions which protect the inner vulva. The inner lips or *labia minora*, are thin and hairless and usually fit inside the labia majora, although it is perfectly normal for them to protrude in some women. The labia minora contain the glands which secrete lubricating juice when you are sexually aroused. If you follow the labia minora up towards your tummy with your finger, you will see that they join together just above the *clitoris*, partly surrounding the clitoris to form its hood. Here you may see or feel the clitoris protruding like a small pink knob from beneath its hood. If you stroke it gently you will find your clitoris to be very sensitive and it will send pleasant feelings around the whole of your vulva, perhaps making you feel a bit 'wet' or aroused. Many women find direct stimulation of the clitoris painful or uncomfortable; this is also quite normal and you may find you prefer gentle stroking over the hood of your clitoris, over your knickers or some other movement where you are in control of the pressure or where the clitoris is touched indirectly.

Just inside the inner lips is a deep area called the *vestibule* which contains glands that produce lubricant for the vulva. Unfortunately not much else is known about the function of this area as we shall see later. Within the vestibule there are two small openings: the small one just below your clitoris is your *urethra*, where urine comes out; below this is the larger opening of the *vagina*. Seeing how close together these two entrances are may help you to understand why many women experience urinary tract infections after having sex. Inside the vagina are fleshy vaginal walls which feel warm and moist. These walls contain pelvic floor muscles which can be contracted and released voluntarily by holding yourself in as you do when you are trying not to pee. Below the vaginal opening where the labia meet is a small area of usually hairless skin called the *perineum*, which goes down towards your anus. It is the perineum which is often torn or cut during childbirth in order for the baby to pass through more easily. If you slide your finger into your vagina pointing towards the small of your back, you may pass over a hard ridge which is the bottom of the *cervix*. It is through here that your menstrual flow passes from the *uterus* to the vagina and it is also through here that the sperm must swim, from the vagina into the uterus and then into the *fallopian tubes* to fertilize an egg to make you pregnant.

Vulval and Vaginal Health

If you are experiencing pain around or just inside the entrance of the vagina, this could be a sign of a dry vagina, an infection which should be treated, a skin problem or an indication of an allergic reaction which can be easily cleared up. For all conditions affecting the vagina and vulva (*see fig. 1*) it is best to consult your doctor, or preferably to visit a clinic that specializes in sexually transmitted diseases. In Britain, these clinics are called genito-urinary medicine (GUM) clinics, sexual health, or sexual medicine clinics, and they are usually part of your local hospital. These clinics are specifically geared up to deal with all aspects of sexual health and most of the tests are done at the hospital straight away so you can get the correct treatment quickly. They are free on the NHS and the service is totally confidential.

The difficulty with many of the conditions described below is that they blur the ridiculously rigid demarcations between gynaecology, urology, genito-urinary medicine, psychology and general practice. You may have to see doctors in more than one of these areas to get a diagnosis, but ensure that you consult as many people as possible to get satisfactory advice.

Regardless of which medical practitioner you visit, it is likely that he or she will probably give you an internal examination. Even though you may prefer to get a diagnosis simply by describing your symptoms to the doctor, the internal examination is vital if your symptoms require a thorough examination and tests. Some women dread this experience, finding it demeaning and painful. These feelings can deter some women from seeking important medical help. If you are nervous, let the doctor know how you feel. Ask him/her what the procedure is before you undress, as once you've got no clothes on and are lying down you are physically more vulnerable and information is harder to take in. Talking about your anxiety may help to alleviate it and breathing deeply will always help you relax. If you practise the sensations at home by gently inserting a clean finger into the vagina in you own time you may feel less anxious. Remember you are not alone, many women find internals unpleasant, but in reality the internal examination is quick and only slightly uncomfortable if the doctor is experienced, and it is in your own interests to undergo it. Although this is generally the case, undergoing an internal examination can be problematic if you are suffering from vestibulitis or vaginismus. However, there are ways to deal with this which I will explain later in the chapter. You can ask for a female doctor to conduct the examination if this makes you more comfortable; if so, it is best to make your request when you actually book the appointment.

What Does the Internal Examination Involve?

You may find it easier to wear a skirt to the appointment if you think you are going to have an internal examination, as you will simply have to remove your knickers and lift your skirt up to your thighs, instead of stripping off from the waist down. Again, GUM clinics are totally geared up for this and you will have somewhere to undress in private and a place to put your belongings. When you are comfortable, the doctor will look inside your vagina by first inserting a well-lubricated metal or plastic speculum into your vagina, then will gently open up the blades of the speculum.

PAINFUL SEX

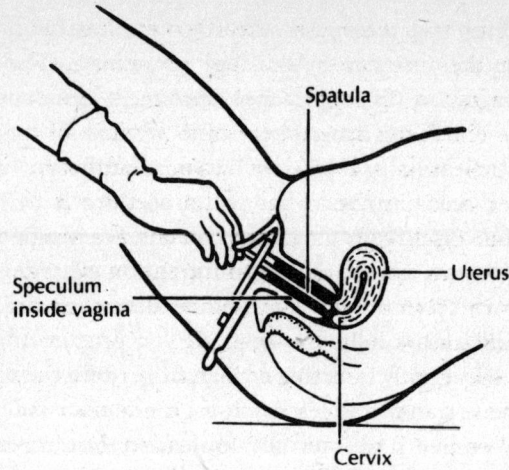

Figure 2

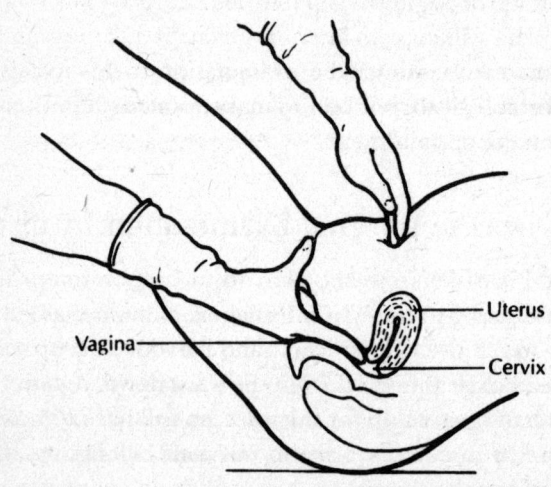

Figure 3

VAGINAL INFECTIONS AND IRRITATIONS

If you have ever had a cervical smear (or pap test) you will be familiar with the instrument and the procedure. The blades stretch the vaginal walls slightly and hold them open, enabling the doctor to check the appearance of the walls and the cervix. At the same time he or she will take swabs, if necessary, by quickly wiping over areas in the vagina, vulva and cervix to pick up samples of your discharge and natural mucus. It is worth remembering that you can ask the doctor to use the smallest speculum, and if you are feeling very sore, express your anxieties and remind the doctor to be especially gentle (*see fig. 2 and 3*).

After the speculum is removed, the doctor will gently insert one or two gloved and lubricated fingers inside your vagina, and using the other hand, will feel the lower abdomen in order to detect any abnormal tenderness, lumps or thickening in the ovaries, tubes and uterus.

Types of Vaginal Infection

All the conditions listed below are vaginal infections which can be detected either by the examination just described or by more specific investigations and tests which are explained under their individual headings.

Vaginal Thrush – Yeast Infection

I got my first bout of thrush (yeast infection) 11 years ago and I have been getting it persistently ever since. Each time I feel so sore and miserable that I'll do anything to avoid catching it. It does put me off sex and sometimes I find it hard to get aroused. But I find I'm less likely to get an attack if a condom is used and I wash without soap before and after sex.

SUSAN, 47

PAINFUL SEX

I experience terrible itching and soreness from thrush (yeast infection) which I have had on and off now for three years. Last summer I seemed to have it for three months constantly. Whenever there is a weakness in my body, or I am stressed it appears, which makes my health even worse. I feel sexual but I don't feel very appealing because I've got this recurring infection. I do enjoy sex but it's always in the back of my mind that I will get it again afterwards and I get embarrassed about oral sex as I'm worried he might be able to taste it.

LORRAINE, 27

How Do You Know If You Have Thrush?

Thrush is extremely common. It is estimated that 75 per cent of women world-wide suffer from it at some point in their lives. Thrush is most commonly caused by an organism called *Candida albicans* that normally lives quite harmlessly on your skin, and in your mouth and gut. It is actually a type of yeast. Under certain conditions, the candida grows and multiplies in the genital areas of both men and women. This overgrowth of candida often results in a white cottage-cheese type of vaginal discharge which causes redness, soreness and itching around your vagina, vulva and sometimes the anus. As the area is sore, you will probably experience pain when you have sex and when you urinate.

What Causes It?

You are more likely to get thrush if you are:

- Pregnant.
- Taking certain antibiotics.
- Diabetic.
- Run down or ill.
- Wearing tight jeans or nylon underwear.
- Having sex with someone who has thrush.
- Anaemic.

Any of the above can trigger an episode of thrush, but it can also result from taking antibiotics that wipe out not only the particular bacteria that is causing your infection, but also other helpful bacteria which normally keep the yeast balance in your vagina in check. Recent research has shown that you are five and half times more likely to develop thrush following antibiotic treatment. The risk varies according to the antibiotic[1] – Keflex, Zinnat and Velosef carry the highest risk, with Bactrim and Septrin carrying the lowest. Some doctors believe that thrush may also be linked to the use of some oral contraceptive pills as these alter the natural pH balance of the vagina; other doctors believe that this theory has been outdated by the introduction of more sophisticated pills which do not have such a strong effect on the hormone balance.

What Can Be Done?

To test for thrush, the doctor will wipe a swab over your vulva and inside the vagina. The swab is sent away for a 'culture test' to see if *Candida albicans* is present. Discharge and itchiness are also symptoms of other infections such as bacterial vaginosis (*see pages 15 – 17*) and it is important that a diagnosis is not made just by looking or describing the symptoms.

Treatment for thrush is relatively easy; usually an anti-fungal cream and pessaries such as Canesten or Nystatin are prescribed. The pessary is an almond-shaped tablet which a woman inserts high up into her vagina with a special applicator. The applicator is similar to the tube that slide some types of tampons into place. The pessaries are only used at night when you are prone, so that the treatment does not spill out. You can use the treatment while you are having a period, since these products are inserted when you are horizontal and relatively motionless, but do not use tampons at any time during this treatment because they will soak up the medication. Oils in the pessaries tend to weaken the latex of condoms and diaphragms, so do not rely on these for contraception. You should wait three days after medication ends to allow all traces of the medication to be either absorbed or discharged before using condoms or a diaphragm again. Up to 10 per cent of women may be allergic to Canesten, and in these cases other anti-fungal medications can be used. Ketoconazole (Nizoral), an anti-fungal medication which also has anti-inflammatory properties has been shown to be effective; in capsule form, it is taken orally.

Oral capsules represent the newest form of treatment and are far more convenient to use. Some oral treatments require only a single dose and can be taken immediately, whereas you must wait until bedtime to use a pessary as this sort of treatment works best when you are prone. Oral treatments can also be used during a period, and as there is no mess involved, you may be able to resume sexual activity more readily. Oral treatment, however, is not suitable for pregnant women.

Although, as explained earlier, the pill is unlikely to be the cause of thrush, Dr White at the Heartlands Hospital in Birmingham has observed that changing from an oestrogen-balanced pill to a progesterone-balanced pill can sometimes reduce the recurrence of thrush. Some women cease being affected by recurrent thrush after going on the progesterone-only pill (the mini pill)[2], or Depo Provera[3], the injectable contraceptive. But one side-effect of these two contraceptives is infrequent or no periods.

Complementary Therapy

Some women have benefited from using plain live yoghurt on the affected area as this contains *lactobacilli* which can help restore the floral balance of the vagina and can also help to soothe the irritation. This is easily done by using a tampon with an applicator. Push the tampon down inside the applicator tube, without letting it fall out, then top up the tube with yoghurt, preferably chilled from the fridge. Insert the tampon into your vagina pushing the yoghurt in with it. The tampon can then be removed. Many women find that eating live yoghurt or taking *acidophilus* tablets (available from health shops or chemists) can help to protect against thrush. A specialist at the Long Island Jewish Medical Centre in America found that when a number of women with recurrent thrush ate live yoghurt daily, they were found to have a *threefold* decrease in infections[4].

DIET

Some complementary therapists believe that persistent vaginal thrush (yeast infection) is a result of an overgrowth of *Candida albicans* in the small intestine, and that dramatically reducing the yeast-feeding foods in our diet will bring this overgrowth under control. Eliminating foods such as sugar, mushrooms, bread, citrus fruit, dairy products, alcohol and processed drinks from the diet is seen to be a crucial part of candida control and numerous books have been written on the subject. But beware of therapists who suggest this is the only cure. The diet suggested is very rigorous and hard to stick to for a lengthy period of time (I have failed in all my attempts). It is also worth bearing in mind that two medical studies which have used yeast-killing Nystatin tablets as a way of reducing candida in the gut have shown that this has little or no effect on recurrent attacks of vaginal thrush. But a change in diet may work by improving local immunity, so it is worth trying for three months to see if there is any improvement.

Garlic is an anti-fungal food and a natural antibiotic. Some women find inserting a clove into the vagina can relieve thrush. Slice a clove in half, wrap in some gauze, insert just at the entrance of the vagina and leave overnight. Do not forget to take it out. Freeze dried garlic supplements and a diet high in fresh garlic have also been known to help some candida sufferers.

AROMATHERAPY

Some women have benefited from adding 2–5 drops of essential oil to their bath; lavender, tea tree and juniper are thought to be the most effective.

Herbal Treatments

Calendula (pot marigold) is an anti-fungal and anti-inflammatory herb ideal for treating thrush. You can buy calendula cream over the counter in most leading chemists or health stores, or you can make your own ointment by adding 5 drops of tea tree essential oil and 5 drops marigold essential oil to a 60g ointment base. Golden seal is a traditional healing herb of native American Indians. Bathe or douche the infected area using 5ml golden seal tincture to 100ml water. Herbalists also cite Aloe vera gel as an anti-fungal; it can also be used to soothe thrush, but it needs to be as pure as possible.

Recurrent Thrush

Thrush can become a real nuisance and cause untold misery when it keeps recurring, especially since it is difficult to tell if repeated attacks are due to reinfection or simply the original infection which has not gone away.

The strict definition of recurrent thrush is six or more attacks a year, where the thrush gets better and comes back. If you are not on the pill and get recurrent thrush, you can take preventive action by using a Canesten pessary on day 10 of your cycle, as day 12 (around the time of ovulation) seems to be a period of reoccurrence. Use one again on day 18 since day 21 (just before your period) is also a risky time. Alternatively you can take pessaries or oral treatments once a month to see if this stops recurrence. Make sure you are checked regularly and do not diagnose yourself as the symptoms of thrush (yeast infection) can also be the symptoms for other vaginal infections such as chlamydia, vestibulitis and bacterial vaginosis. Persistent thrush can also be a sign of diabetes or anaemia and it is worth eliminating these conditions as the possible cause. Some women find relief from recurrent thrush (yeast infection) with a course of iron tablets. Some doctors believe that if you have chronic itching but not necessarily discharge and a positive culture test, it could be because you are allergic to *Candida albicans*. Unfortunately, research into this area is not yet conclusive but the symptoms can be relieved by taking regular saltwater baths, which kill off excess yeast, and the application of a mild steroid cream to relieve the itching. Candida can also live in the gut and the anus, and as pessaries only kill the overgrowth in the vagina it is possible that you may find oral treatments which kill excess candida in the gut, anus and vagina more effective.

Chronic Thrush

A small minority of thrush attacks may be due to another type of yeast called *Candida galbrata* which does not respond well to the usual treatments. Anti-fungal treatments such as Gyno-Daktarin or Gyno Pervaryl are useful for chronic thrush.

Prevention

The reason you may suffer repeated attacks after intercourse may not be due to reinfection via your partner, but because you are stirring up candida that has bored itself into the membranes of the vagina. This can be avoided by making sure you are fully aroused and lubricated before allowing your partner to penetrate you; if need be, lots of lubricant can lend a helping hand. An ideal method would be using Canesten cream as a lubricant to keep the thrush in check. If possible, have a saltwater bath after sex. It is easy to trace whether your partner is reinfecting you or not simply by using condoms for a few months to see whether the attacks stop. If the attacks do stop, then it would be wise for your partner to be examined and treated before you stop using condoms. Men may suffer similar symptoms to women, these include irritation, burning or itching under the foreskin, discharge under the foreskin, and redness or red patches in this area.

It is important to note that you can get reinfected from a sexual partner who may not have any symptoms. Anal sex is best avoided if you have recurrent thrush (yeast infection) as this could cause thrush to be transferred from the anus to the vagina. Dr Morrison at the GUM clinic in Freedom Fields Hospital, Plymouth, recommends that women with thrush wash their knickers with non-biological powder, rinse them thoroughly and then iron the crotch area when dry to kill off any remaining candida spores.

Thrush and Cystitis

Cystitis is an inflammation of the bladder which is normally caused by bacteria. Symptoms are most commonly a feeling of urgency to urinate and pain when passing water (*see page 20 for further description*). Many women experience cystitis-like symptoms when they have thrush and vice versa. This may be because the yeast that irritates the vagina can also irritate the area where you urinate from (the urethra) and the bladder. (One way to avoid this 'double whammy' is to have a saltwater bath after sex, as this will kill off any bacteria and excess yeast.) Another reason is that one of the trigger factors for thrush is the use of antibiotics, and these are often prescribed for cystitis. To avoid this, ensure you get thrush treatments – preferably oral ones – at the same time as you receive antibiotics, and use them preventatively.

Trichomoniasis Vaginalis

Also known as TV, this sexually transmitted disease is caused by a parasite that literally swims into the vaginal mucus, usually as a result of unprotected intercourse. Once infected, it usually takes about a week or two for the symptoms to show. The most notable symptom is usually a yellow-green coloured foamy discharge with an unpleasant odour. The vulva is usually sore and red, and during

VAGINAL INFECTIONS AND IRRITATIONS

an attack you will probably find penetration too painful to consider. You may also experience burning when you urinate, similar to cystitis. Men often experience no symptoms, but some men do suffer pain when passing urine and have a discharge from the penis.

Treatment

The treatment for TV is a five- to seven-day course of antibiotics such as Flagyll which must be taken by you and your partner. No alcohol or sex until you are cured! It is wise to be checked again after treatment, as it can recur in rare cases. If this happens, a longer course of treatment is necessary.

Prevention

A good preventive available from the chemist is Aci-gel, a product which is helpful in maintaining the pH balance of the vagina by improving the acid balance. However, it can cause further irritation; stop using it immediately if this happens.

In a study of nearly 500 men at the University of Washington School of Medicine in Seattle, *trichomonaisis* was found in nearly 25 per cent of the men whose partners were diagnosed with the infection and in 6 per cent of randomly selected heterosexual men. Consequently, if you have TV your sexual partner should also be tested and treated to avoid passing it back and forth between you. If you feel you may be at risk, use a condom. It has also been noted that TV can be passed on through the use of sex toys such as vibrators. Make sure that these are throroughly clean before use and don't share them with a partner.

Bacterial Vaginosis

This is an increasingly common condition which in 1990 accounted for 33 per cent of all vaginal infections seen at GUM clinics in Britain[5]. In hospital trials in Britain and America some doctors have observed that bacterial vaginosis (BV) is more common than thrush (yeast infection) but is often mistaken for it. But unlike thrush, if BV is left untreated it can wreak havoc. The symptoms of BV are:

- Thin white or grey discharge which sticks to the sides of the vagina.
- Musty odour, especially after sex or periods.
- Itching and burning of the vagina and vulva which makes sex painful for one-third of sufferers.

The cause of BV is still a mystery, but basically, the normal vaginal ecosystem is thrown out of synch and the normal flora are replaced by hostile bacteria. About 15 types of bacteria normally live in the vagina, and in healthy women, one species – *lactobacillus* – predominates, accounting for 90 per cent of the organisms there. Lactobacillus fights infection by producing lactic acid and hydrogen peroxide to repel harmful bacteria. Bacterial vaginosis occurs when the lactobacillus is wiped out, allowing the 'bad bacteria' to take over. It is not considered to be sexually transmitted although sexual activity or other genital infections can trigger it, as they naturally disrupt the vaginal ecosystem. BV infection has nothing to do with hygiene, and women who think they are unclean and treat a suspected infection by douching or excessive washing may make the infection worse, or themselves more prone to infection. As the symptoms of burning and itching are similar to thrush, you must go to the doctor for tests rather than diagnose it yourself. The doctor will take samples of the discharge and vaginal fluid and send them for laboratory analysis to see if your infection is BV or thrush.

It is particularly important to test for BV if you have any symptoms when you are pregnant or about to undergo gynaecological surgery, because during these times it can cause dangerous complications such as premature labour or a risk of pelvic

VAGINAL INFECTIONS AND IRRITATIONS

inflammatory disease (*see page 65*)[6]. After giving birth, women who have BV are six times more likely to develop endometriosis (*see page 75*)[7]. Because of the particular risks for pregnant women, doctors such as Dr Phillip Hay from St George's Hospital, London, argue that all pregnant women should be screened. In his survey 15 per cent of the pregnant women screened were found to have bacterial vaginosis in early pregnancy. These women had a fivefold increased risk of late miscarriage or pre-term delivery. If you are thinking about getting pregnant, or are pregnant and have noticed an unusual discharge, you may like to have a test.

Treatment

Two antibiotics that work well for BV are Metronidazole and Clindamycin. The average cure rate after this treatment is around 80 per cent. Meteronidazole does have side-effects, including nausea and headaches, and pregnant women cannot take it. Topical versions of successful antibiotics have recently been developed and can be used safely by pregnant women. The cream is usually applied to the vagina once daily, before bed for seven nights[8].

Complementary Therapy

Lactic acid pessaries used to be the common complementary therapy treatment for vaginosis but recent trials have found them to be ineffectual. An Israeli study recently showed that the yoghurt tampon treatment as described earlier for thrush (yeast infection) was extremely effective in treating BV in pregnant women.

Prevention

Some correlation has been found between the recurrence of BV and use of the contraceptive sponge, perhaps because the sponge can harbour the harmful bacteria. If you suffer from an attack, it may be wise to switch to condoms or some other birth control method.

Chlamydia

Until recently this condition has been little understood and little recognized, but the incidence of chlamydia has increased dramatically over the recent decade and is now the most common sexually transmitted disease in the world. It is caused by a bacteria, yet it behaves like a virus, hiding in the cells of the cervix. Consequently, 70 per cent of infected women and 25 per cent of infected men have no symptoms[9]. The symptoms to look for in women are:

- Abnormal vaginal discharge.
- Pain on passing urine.
- Abdominal pain.
- Pain *during* sexual intercourse.
- Bleeding between periods, after sex, or heavier than normal periods.
- Pain or cramps in the stomach or lower back, *particularly after sex.*

The symptoms to look for in men are:

- Pain on urination.
- Discharge from the penis.
- Inflammation of rectum and anus.

Chlamydia is particularly common in young women and those under 35 are seen to be at the highest risk. Prevalence studies in GP[10] and gynaecology clinics in Britain show that up to 12 per cent of women in this age group could be infected. American studies are even more alarming. The Center for Disease Control and Prevention predicted 4 million new cases in the USA for 1994 and estimated that 50,000 women would be left sterile as a result. Unfortunately, women are much more at risk than men. In the USA, a woman's chance of contracting chlamydia in a single act of unprotected sex is 40 per cent, twice that of a man.

The chlamydia infection hides in the cells in the cervix (the neck of the womb) and, if it is not treated, the fallopian tubes can become inflamed and blocked. This infection may spread to the ovaries and womb causing abdominal pain, and may lead to pelvic inflammatory disease (*see page 65*). Chlamydia is currently thought to be a major contributing factor in around 60 per cent of pelvic inflammatory disease cases. It is associated with up to half of all cases of cervicitis, an inflammation of the cervix which can cause bleeding after sex and an offensive discharge.

Diagnosis involves looking for the antibodies for chlamydia using a variety of methods. Cell culture, which involves taking a swab from the cervix, is the most common way. Once the diagnosis has been confirmed, the treatment for chlamydia is simple; a course of tetracycline or erythromycin antibiotics is prescribed. It is vital that the course is completed and that you abstain from sex for two weeks to give the area time to heal. Chlamydia often manifests itself in men as non-specific urethritis (NSU) or non-gonocchal urethritis (NGU) and consequently, if your partner has suffered from this very common condition, it is important that you be checked for chlamydia.

New tests that detect chlamydia in men's urine are being developed; they will make it easier to screen sexually active men, who now have to undergo a painful urethral swab, and research is also being done on a urine test for women. Also just introduced is a new treatment for men and women which involves a single oral dose of antibiotics, instead of a seven-day regime which can be hard to maintain.

Prevention

Research has shown that women who use the contraceptive cap or diaphragm (which helps protect the cervix), are around 70 per cent less likely to contract chlamydia[11]; condom use also significantly reduces the risk. As chlaymdial infections are so common and often do not show symptoms, it is advisable to go for regular check-ups to ensure the absence or rapid treatment of these infections, especially if you are pregnant, or planning a baby. If your smear test shows up 'inflammation' on the cervix, this could be due to chlamydia and it is worth going for a screening. Some doctors, alarmed by the recent increase in this condition, are pressing for widespread general screening for chlamydia.

Cystitis – Urinary Tract Infections

Like thrush (yeast infection), cystitis is so common that women are often expected to live with it as they would with a common cold, and yet it causes a great deal of depression and anguish. Nearly half of all women in the UK will get a painful attack of cystitis at sometime in their lives[12]. These attacks are most common among women in their late teens and twenties when they are most sexually active, and at the menopause, when the mucous lining of the vagina becomes dry.

The urinary tract consists of the kidneys, ureters, bladder and urethra. Liquid containing nutrients and waste products is filtered from the blood by the kidneys and passes down the ureters to the bladder as urine. The urine eventually passes out of the body through the urethra. Normally the urine contains some bacteria but it is only when bacteria multiply in the urine that a urinary infection occurs. Because a woman's urinary tract is close to the anus and vagina, it is often more susceptible than a man's to infections. If it is confined to the bladder, it is known as cystitis. The symptoms of cystitis are:

VAGINAL INFECTIONS AND IRRITATIONS

- Unusually frequent desire to pass urine, often only a little (or none) is passed.
- Stinging and burning sensations during the passing of urine.
- Burning sensations at the outer end of the urethra, extending to the vagina.
- Urine has a strong odour.
- Urine contains blood in more severe cases.
- Abdominal pain, back pain and feeling feverish.

Women more commonly suffer from urinary infections than men as they have a shorter urethra, which means that bacteria from the vagina or anus has a shorter distance to travel. Sexual intercourse or vaginal stimulation can account for some attacks of cystitis. The urethra is just above the vagina and sexual activity can massage bacteria from the vagina, the anus or surrounding area, into the urethra and up into the bladder. Cystitis can also occur if the bladder or urethra are prone to irritation from substances such as alcohol or spicy food. Cystitis is usually treated with antibiotics which will kill off the bacteria causing the infection. For this reason, a urine sample needs to be taken and cultured to determine which antibiotic will be most effective. You will need to provide a urine sample as soon as the first signs occur, so make an appointment with your doctor promptly.

You could take a urine sample yourself:

1 Use a sterile urine sample bottle which you can get from a chemist. If you do not have one, wash a clean glass jar thoroughly with very hot water and detergent, then rinse with boiling water.
2 Take a sample of your urine midway through your pee. This is called a mid-stream sample.
3 Write your name, your doctor's name and the date on a sticky label and place it on the bottle. Store the bottle in the fridge until you can see your doctor.

If laboratory analysis reveals that there are red or white blood cells in the urine, then you have an infection. However, it takes about three days to determine whether bacteria is present, so in the meantime you could try to relieve your suffering by following the measures below and taking some painkillers. Some doctors will prescribe one of a number of antibiotics most likely to clear the infection before the results of tests arrive and will change them if necessary when the results come back. The antibiotics are taken over a three- to five-day period combined with a high fluid intake (about four pints a day).

Non-Bacterial Cystitis

If you have tried all the self-help measures and are still getting persistent symptoms without evidence of infection, you may be suffering from interstitial cystitis (*see page 42*). Not maintaining a sufficient intake of water-based liquids allows the bladder and urethra to become dry and leads to crystals of the uric acid irritating the delicate tissue. Jeans with their tight knot of seam which bruises the urethral opening; clothes which restrict air access such as tight trousers, leotards, lycra exercise wear, tights and swimming costumes full of salt and sand can all be a source of irritation. If no infection is found then your cystitis may have another cause other than infection. It can be caused by a variety of factors including poor hygiene, perfumed toiletries or, most commonly, deydration.

Complementary Therapy

HOMOEOPATHY
Offers a range of remedies for cystitis. *Apis mel* is recommended if there is a burning sensation when passing urine. Take *Cantharsis* if there is an overwhelming urge to urinate with little results. *Pulsatilla* should be taken if your symptoms feel worse when lying down and urine is accidentally passed when coughing or passing wind.

VAGINAL INFECTIONS AND IRRITATIONS

HERBALISM
Diuretic herbal teas such as chamomile, couch grass or marshmallow can also be useful. Supplements of propolis, a natural antibiotic made from honey, may be useful in eliminating harmful bacteria.

AROMATHERAPY
Make a massage oil from 20–25 ml soya oil and 5 drops of either cajuput, niaouli, parsley, pine or sandalwood and massage into the hands, feet, tummy and lower back.

Cranberry Juice

Cranberry juice has also been found to be an effective preventive and treatment for cystitis. Israeli researchers discovered that it contains a compound which prevents the offending bacteria from attaching itself to the bladder. A large glass of cranberry juice daily can act as a preventive; according to research in the *Journal of the American Medical Association*[13], the fruit inhibits the growth of *E. coli* bacteria. In this trial, 60 post-menopausal women at risk of urinary infections drank 300 ml of cranberry juice a day for a period of six months, while a control group of 61 post-menopausal women drank a cranberry juice lookalike. After just one month of juice drinking, researchers found only 15 per cent of the cranberry group had infected urine compared with 28 per cent in the control group – an improvement which continued until the end of the trial. And women in the cranberry group who did develop urinary infections were far more likely to fight the infection off than the others.

The secret of the cranberry's success lies in two vital ingredients: fructose, which is common to most fruits, and an antibacterial compound, also contained in blueberries, which apparently helps to stop *E. coli* bacteria from sticking to the urinary tract wall.

Prevention

Persistent cystitis can often be completely cleared up by strict adherence to self-help measures. At the first early signs of an attack make sure you do a sample straight away as then it is far easier for the doctor to find out if there is an infection present. If you get recurrent attacks, ensure you have a couple of sterile bottles from your doctor in stock for emergencies. After this drink a pint of water mixed with a teaspoon of bicarbonate of soda which acts to neutralize the urine and stop it from burning. Or you can use one of several over-the-counter preparations, such as Cymalon, which are available from chemists. Avoid tea, coffee and alcohol. And be aware that long, hot soaks in the bath can cause attacks in some women. Swab the urethral area with cotton wool made moist with cool water, to calm the inflammation.

Cystitis attacks have been connected to some contraceptive methods. Some women have found that substituting the pill, which sometimes creates extra mucus that can irritate the urethra, for another form of contraceptive, lessens the attacks. Other women are allergic to spermicidal creams or lubricants. If the contraceptive cap or diaphragm are left in for a long time, or not washed properly between insertions, they can act as a reservoir for bacteria. If the cap is too large, it may press against the urethra, causing cystitis-like symptoms. A general rule is also to empty the bladder when you need to keep the system going and don't hold it in. You can also take the following steps before and after sex to avoid getting an attack. Although some of these procedures may rule out spontaneity, then so does cystitis!

BEFORE SEX

You and your partner should wash your genital and anal areas, and hands to avoid the transmission of bacteria. Check the area under the foreskin to make sure it is clean. If your bladder or bowels are full, empty them. Vibrators and other sex toys should also be washed beforehand and used with care. If you have anal sex, use a condom and change it before penetrating the vagina and use a lubricant such as KY Jelly, if necessary, for both vaginal and anal penetration.

After Sex

Pass urine immediately after intercourse, even if it is just a small bit in order to flush out any bacteria which may have travelled up the urethra. Pour cool water from a bottle over the vaginal area and gently pat yourself dry. Drink three of four glasses of water and try to empty your bladder before going to sleep.

Sometimes what may appear to be recurrent cystitis could be a sexually transmitted disease such as chlamydia. If this is suspected, then a vaginal swab for culturing should be taken by a doctor.

Food Irritants

Concentrated fruit juices are very acidic and can produce acidic urine which irritates the urethra. Spicy foods such as pepper, vinegar, pickles and curry powder can also irritate the bladder.

Herpes Simplex

The word 'herpes' has unfortunately become a loaded term and people with herpes have been made to feel stigmatized, ashamed or unclean. This is unfair, unfounded and discriminatory – no one can be 'blamed' for herpes simplex and having it says nothing about your personal hygiene. Many doctors feel that the implications of genital herpes simplex have been dramatically over-sensationalized in terms of the threat it poses to your general health. It is a relatively harmless, low-grade virus, as common as chicken pox, and almost everyone will come into contact with it, at some time, with or without symptoms. Marian Covey from the Herpes Association believes that the real suffering is not caused solely by the discomfort of the condition but by the psychological effect of the stigma which has been attached to herpes simplex.

What Is It?

Herpes simplex is a virus which exists in two main types. Type one typically causes the recurrent cold sores some people suffer around the mouth. Type two is found to cause recurrent symptoms on the genitals. However, both types of herpes can exist at both sites. Over half of the people affected do not experience recurrent symptoms even though they may carry the virus and shed it from time to time. The symptoms in women are:

- Flu-like symptoms and sometimes bowel and stomach disorders.
- Tingly or itchy sensation around the vagina and vulva.
- Pain when urinating, as the urine may flow over the sores.
- Pain when sitting or walking.
- Swelling of lymph glands in the groin.
- Small red spots on the vulva, vagina, urethra, cervix and sometimes the anus. These spots turn into small, sometimes painful blisters which may burst, leaving small red ulcers, which on 'dry' skin (not the vulva, labia, inside the vagina or cervix), form a hard crust. These clear up in seven to twelve days.

Recurrent symptoms rarely involve flu-like sensations and all other symptoms are generally minor in comparison with the primary, or first, occurrence.

Transmission can happen through body contact and friction with herpes simplex lesions on fingers, mouth or genitals. Once the lesions have healed and become crusted over, they are no long infectious. Unfortunately, herpes simplex can recur, but at intervals varying from a few weeks to several years apart. Because people who have had one occurrence will have developed some antibodies to it, a recurrence is almost always less severe, with far fewer lesions and is generally localized to a single area. In women, this will usually be on visible parts of the body such as the outer labia (the hairy lips), the groin or tops of the thighs.

Treatment

Your doctor may be able to tell whether you have herpes simplex just by examining the affected area. In some cases a swab of the spots may be taken to confirm the diagnosis. Like chicken pox or flu and other viruses, symptoms of herpes simplex are naturally cured by the body's natural defences. An oral dose of Acyclovir (Zovirax) five times a day for five days has been shown to reduce a recurrent episode by a day but it does not help the pain or itching. A local anaesthetic ointment such as Xylocaine is far more effective for this and it has been shown in one study[14] that this ointment can prevent recurrence in 50 per cent of genital cases.

Canadian doctors have had great success using liquid nitrogen to freeze the lesions. The liquid nitrogen is applied with a cotton-tipped applicator to the affected area, no matter how extensive, to freeze the entire thickness of the lesions. It provides great pain relief and the sores disappear rapidly[15].

Complementary Therapy

HOMOEOPATHY

Some people have found homoeopathic remedies to be helpful – particularly *Nat Mur* and *Rhus Tox*.

HERBALISM

Recently, echinea, a blood purifying plant has been found to be effective with herpes simplex. Take one capsule three times a day or make a soothing tea and take three cups a day for a month.

AROMATHERAPY

Success has been reported using diluted tea tree essential oil on the affected area. The Herpes Association reports that many members have found this treatment to be particularly helpful. Well-known aromatherapist Robert Tisserand recommends diluted rose otto essential oil, applied directly to the lesions but not the surrounding skin. Unfortunately this oil is very expensive.

Prevention

There many things you can do at the first sign of a herpes recurrence to inhibit it from developing further. The Herpes Association in Britain suggests the following:

- Keep the area as cool as possible. Apply ice-cubes in a plastic bag or wrapped in a handkerchief for ten minutes at a time if possible.
- Spend half an hour with your feet up, fully relaxing and ensure you get adequate sleep. Be kind to yourself.

Risks of catching genital herpes simplex can be reduced if condoms (male or female) are used, although there is still a risk if sores are outside the protected genital area.

How To Avoid Spreading Herpes Simplex

While you have active facial herpes simplex do not kiss anyone anywhere on the body unless you know they have also had active symptoms. Do not have sexual intercourse, give or receive oral sex when you have active genital herpes simplex – this applies from the first signs of tingling until the lesions have healed completely.

Remember you cannot *reinfect* yourself or your partner. This is all you have to remember – simple straightforward precautions. If you get it into perspective, herpes simplex should play a minor part in your sex life. It is not necessary to tell everyone concerned about your herpes unless you are in a sexual situation while you have active sores; you do not ask a partner if he or she has ever had a coldsore before you kiss them – it is the same thing with herpes simplex!

Genital Herpes Simplex and Pregnancy

A few powerful myths, unfortunately still propagated by some misguided doctors need to be dispelled here. Your unborn baby is only at risk of contracting the virus if you have your *first* episode of genital herpes simplex in the last few weeks of pregnancy. This is extremely rare, but if this did occur, there is a risk that the baby could pick up the virus on the way down the birth canal. Only in this case would a caesarean section be justifiable.

Genital Warts and Human Papilloma Virus

As you probably know, warts are small, fleshy growths on the skin that can appear almost anywhere on the body. They are caused by a virus called the human papilloma virus (HPV) of which there are around 70 different strains. When warts appear on the genitals, they are, quite naturally, called genital warts.

You can catch HPV if you have skin-to-skin contact with the wart virus. This does not necessarily mean that you have to have penetrative sex with a man with genital warts to catch the virus, as is still commonly thought. The wart virus can also be passed on through non-penetrative sex, finger foreplay and oral sex which means that lesbians and women who have safe, protected penetrative sex are, unfortunately, still at risk.

Symptoms

In women genital warts are found in the vulva, vagina, cervix and anus. You might see them or feel them, or your partner might notice them. They can be small, flat smooth bumps, or quite large, pink, cauliflower-like bumps. The warts can appear on their own or in groups and can cause itchiness and irritation. It is usually easier to spot warts on a penis than on female genitalia, so if your partner is a man, check regularly for any of these symptoms appearing on him.

You can have the wart virus for months, or even years, before developing warts. Either of you may have got the virus from another sexual partner before you started having sex together. Once you have the virus, it can live on you and be passed to other people for some time. It can be passed on even before the warts are noticeable or after they have disappeared, although doctors agree that you are most infectious when warts are visible. In all cases, the absence of warts is no guarantee that you are not carrying the virus.

Treatment

Genital warts can be treated and removed by a variety of methods. The most common treatment involves painting the wart with a liquid called podophyllin. This is usually done by the doctor in the surgery and you may need to have the treatment two or three times before the wart is fully removed. If it proves to be stubborn, the doctor may try other treatments such as freezing or heating them. Unfortunately, warts can recur so it is vital to keep a regular check.

Prevention

Women are often told that condom use will fully protect them from HPV, but as it can be passed on through any skin-to-skin contact, this is not necessarily true. Obviously, if your partner has genital warts on his penis, it is wise to use a condom to increase your protection. Lesbians should ensure that they go for regular cervical smear tests (pap smears), and challenge any doctor who says this is not necessary as HPV can only be transmitted by heterosexual, penetrative sex. Unfortunately, this view is still common and it is wrong.

HPV Infection

The implications of HPV infection are more important to women than the actual appearance of the warts. This virus has been linked with vulval pain, vulval cancer and an increased risk of cervical cancer, but as yet none of these links have been totally proven and more research needs to be done. Some doctors have found that exposure to HPV on the vulva can result in itching and burning symptoms, but other doctors suggest this is due to reasons other than HPV. There is also concern that women who have been exposed to the wart virus may be at greater risk of cervical cancer. You can prevent this by ensuring that you have regular (yearly) smear or pap tests if you have had warts. Encouragingly, according to a recent report, HPV usually goes away eventually on its own[16].

Chapter 2
NON-INFECTIOUS CAUSES OF VAGINAL PAIN

One of the most common causes of painful intercourse, where a specific infection or bacteria cannot be found, is vaginal dryness, where the vagina is nor lubricating enough. Vulval pain is another cause. As we have seen, the vulva includes the inner and outer labia, the clitoris, the urethra and the entrance to the vagina (*see fig. 1*). Chronic vulval pain involves unexplained burning, itching, throbbing and tenderness if pressure is exerted at any, or all of these sites, which can be anything from a minor annoyance to pain that seriously impinges on your life. As vulval pain has only recently begun to be recognized and understood as a medical condition, the symptoms have been classified under many names depending on the way they manifest themselves and how they respond to treatment. Generalized pain in the area is usually classified as vulvodynia and when the condition has specific sites of soreness, it is usually identified as vulval vestibulitis, or focal vulvitis. The treatments and causes described below are generally applicable to all chronic vulval pain conditions.

NON-INFECTIOUS CAUSES OF VAGINAL PAIN
Vulval Vestibulitis Syndrome

As this condition has only recently been recognized by the medical profession and very little is known about it, I feel that women who have vulval vestibulitis should tell their stories first. Their experiences will shock you.

In 1984 I experienced the most terrible burning sensation at the entrance to my vagina; it was constant and so severe I couldn't lead a normal life. It was like being dipped in acid. My sex life came to a stop as penetration was so painful. The doctors were convinced it was thrush (yeast infection), or all in my head. I was given every ointment and pessary on the market and I had two laporoscopy operations to look around for possible pelvic inflammation, even though this wasn't the source of my pain. I kept telling them it was at the entrance *to my vagina.*

From the beginning I have been treated with disdain by the medical profession. A gynaecologist seen in 1986 could have been helpful as he said he had heard about 'burning vulva syndrome' (now called vestibulitis or vulvodynia) when he was in the USA. But he was obviously cynical about this new syndrome and let me down badly when he sent me to a 'lady' who he said 'would get rid of my symptoms'. I was so pleased that someone would finally cure me, that it took several visits before I realized he'd sent me to a mental hospital for counselling and drugs. Without knowing what they were, I was put on anti-depressants and ended up having sessions with the psychiatrist. This was very distressing and I managed to pluck up the courage to leave before my self-esteem could get any lower. Two years later, I met a doctor who immediately diagnosed vulval vestibulitis. Visiting him was the best decision I've ever made.

MARY, 30

PAINFUL SEX

For the past four years I have suffered from intermittent burning around the vulva. It can clear up for up to two months, during which time sex is possible and then it returns without warning. At the beginning I thought it was thrush (yeast infection) and for the next few months returned to my doctor to be treated for this. But nothing helped and I spent most of 1992 with a bag of frozen peas between my legs! As neither doctors or specialist clinics could find anything wrong I was sent to a sex therapist, but this didn't resolve my very physical pain. I was only 20 and the effects on my sexual identity were devastating. I became paranoid in situations where I might meet men and I was scared if I started to go out with anyone I would have to tell them what was wrong. This led to a virtual disappearance of my sex drive, I considered myself non-sexual, devoid of any sexual needs and incapable of giving.

CLAIRE, 23

What Is Vestibulitis?

In 1983, a group of American doctors set up a working party to study a phenomenon called burning vulva syndrome. They discovered that many women complained of burning, itching, stinging, rawness and pain in that area, causing misery to their lives and preventing them from having sex. Many women had little help from their doctors and some, as we can see above, had even been referred to psychiatrists. Let me state here that this medical ignorance does not mean that this is a new condition, since this syndrome has been described under assorted names over a hundred years ago. As far back as 1889, Dr Skene, in his *Treatise on the Diseases of Women,* described one of the most common disorders of the vulva as 'excessive sensitivity'. He said external manifestations of the disease were lacking, but when 'the examining finger comes in contact with the sensitive part, the patient complains of pain which is sometimes so great as to cause her to cry out'. In 1928, Dr Kelly reported 'exquisitely sensitive deep red spots as a fruitful source of dyspareunia (painful sex)'. Then for more than

NON-INFECTIOUS CAUSES OF VAGINAL PAIN

five decades the medical literature was unaccountably silent on this issue. In 1987, as part of a research team at St Thomas's Hospital in London, the late Dr Friedrich confirmed a collection of symptoms he called 'vulvar vestibulitis syndrome'[1]. These were:

- Severe pain on vaginal entry.
- Tenderness to pressure localized within the vulvar vestibule.
- Redness and inflammation in the area.

The areas most commonly affected are near the bartholins glands at the bottom of the vagina (just above the anus) and the Skene glands either side of the urethra (just under the clitoris), but whether these glands have anything to do with causing the condition is unknown (*see fig. 4*). Friedrich's definition is still not wholly satisfactory as many women suffer the pain constantly regardless of pressure, and it comes and goes spontaneously. Many women report that the pain and soreness is worse around 10 days before menstruation and just after menstruation when the vulva is particularly dry. For some women, almost any pressure is intolerable and they often cannot wear trousers, ride a horse or a bicycle.

What Causes It?

Unfortunately the cause of vestibulitis is still unknown. Biopsies taken from the painful area show non-specific chronic inflammation with no signs of bacteria, viruses or fungi. The following are some current, but still speculative theories.

- Many women who have vulval vestibulitis syndrome (VVS) also suffer from repeated thrush (yeast infection) which has been treated with anti-fungal creams. At first, some doctors thought that an allergy to these might be a factor, but others say that the high incidence of thrush (yeast infection) reported by women at the onset of vulval pain is more likely

Figure 4 — Skene's glands; Bartholin's glands

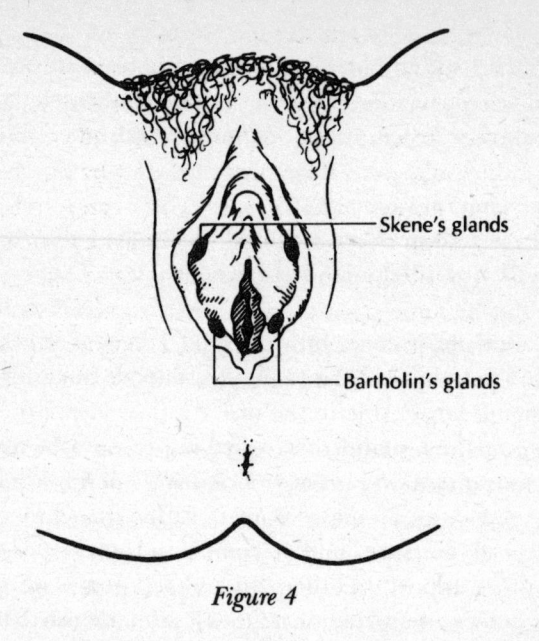

to be an indication of failed diagnosis. Still, there has been much speculation in medical literature about the role of thrush in vulvar vesitibulitis and vulvar pain syndromes.
- Genital warts, caused by the human papilloma virus (HPV) have been found on women with vulvar pain and initially it was thought that the virus was causing the pain. However, genital warts and HPV are also very common in women who experience no vulval pain symptoms.
- Auto-immune factors, where the body attacks itself in a specific area for no obvious reason have been cited by some.

Other theories include hormonal imbalances, genetic predisposition and back problems which can sometimes lead to pain in the vulval area. Both vestibulitis and vulvodynia, which refers to general vulval burning and itching, are called syndromes rather than diseases as no consistent cause has been found.

NON-INFECTIOUS CAUSES OF VAGINAL PAIN

The Oxalate Theory

The Vulval Pain Foundation in America has observed that many women have developed chronic vulval pain after changing to a primarily vegetarian diet, eating more fruit and vegetables which are high in oxalate. Oxalates are produced by organisms in the body during normal metabolism. They can enter the body through digestion of foods containing oxalate and are normally harmlessly excreted from the body as a waste product through urine. But in some cases calcium oxalate can form tiny crystals which cause pain as they make contact with nerve fibres in the body, creating burning and itching sensations in the skin; in this case, the vulval area.

Doctors who tested the urine of one vestibulitis patient over 24 hours found that at certain times of the day her body overproduced calcium oxalate in an erratic, but predictable way, resulting in peaks which usually coincided with her pain[2]. On a low oxalate diet and doses of calcium citrate tablets, which stopped calcium oxalate from forming crystals at her peak overproducing time, this patient was able to become pain-free in about a year.

How Common Is It?

It is very hard to establish real figures for this syndrome because many women are too embarrassed to talk to their doctors about painful sex, and many more are dismissed out of hand if they do not have obvious complaints such as thrush (yeast infection) or BV. But specialists agree that more and more women are coming forward with these symptoms.

One study illustrated the high prevalence of vestibulitis in North America[3]. Dr Goetsch examined all her gynaecological patients over six months for signs of vestibulitis. Out of a total of 210 patients, 31 had the full symptoms. Of these, 15 said they had had pain since they were teenagers. More than half had consulted their doctors about their symptoms and 12 had been told it was thrush (yeast infection).

In Britain, Dr George Morrison, GUM consultant at the Freedom Fields Hospital, Plymouth, Britain, is conducting a study with a local GP to assess the incidence of vestibulitis, but the results are not yet known. What the experts have said is that in their experience, around 98 per cent of women who suffer from vulval vestibulitis are white, heterosexual and premenopausal but whether this is an indication of the syndrome, or a result of social mores and issues around access to health-care is unclear.

Treatment

A wide variety of treatments has been offered to vestibulitis patients but there is still no standard cure. Some women find that their symptoms go away if they stop using bath products, soaps, washing powders or irritant creams on the area. Many women also experience a spontaneous remission from their symptoms for no apparent reason. In other cases, the treatments can be as follows:

- Cortisone creams such as Dermovate ointment for limited periods on the area to reduce inflammation.
- Topical anaesthetics such as 5 per cent Xylocaine ointment can be used to relieve soreness and itching. If applied to the specific areas 15 to 30 minutes prior to lovemaking, it can make sexual stimulation of the clitoris and sexual intercourse pain-free.
- In America, Dr Stanley Marinoff and Dr Maria Turner[4] injected interferon, known for its anti-inflammatory and anti-viral characteristics, directly into the affected area. These injections have been reported to improve the condition considerably in approximately 50 per cent of cases in which they have been tried, but as the injections are directly on the vulva while the patient is awake, they can be painful. More encouraging is the introduction of an interferon cream in the last

six months. Trials to measure its effectiveness on vulvar vestibulitis are being discussed but have yet to be held.
- It is often very hard for a vestibulitis patient to assess whether or not she is 30 or 40 per cent better after treatment. If you had a headache for three years, you probably would not recognize that it was better until the pain had been completely removed. Dr George Morrison and his team at Freedom Fields Hospital in Plymouth have invented a probe machine which can establish the level of discomfort in vulvar vestibulitis patients and this has proven to be a good way of measuring the effectiveness of a treatment objectively. Dr Morrison has found that the tolerance level for pressure on this area in healthy women is between seven and eight, with vestibulitis patients it is around one to four. After treatment with ketoconazole cream (also known as Nizoral) applied three times daily for between four to six months, Dr Morrison has shown that the tolerance level of vestibulitis patients steadily improves.
- Some women have found that Senselle, a vaginal lubricant produced by Durex, soothes the itching and dryness and can help intercourse. A few women have also reported becoming pain-free with regular use. Doctors in America have recently reported successful results with the long-term use of oestrogen creams. It is applied twice daily on the affected area for six months. It is thought that this acts by strengthening the skin and providing it with a better blood supply. It can also be used in conjunction with oxalate therapy (*see below*). Dr Willems, gynaecologist at Scripps Clinic and Research Foundation in La Jolla, California, USA believes that supplemental oestrogen to the vestibule tends to improve the overall resilience of the vulva skin tissue. But he emphasizes that women who benefit from this therapy may not necessarily have a clinical oestrogen deficiency or be menopausal. He uses estradiol 0.01 per cent (brand name

Estrace) but says that there is no reason to believe that other oestrogen creams wouldn't yield the same results. He instructs patients to use approximately the same amount one would put on a toothbrush, twice a day, and to rub it gently into the painful area. The healing process is slow and symptoms may worsen before they get better as the new tissue grows.
- The most drastic solution is surgery where the painful skin is removed and the vagina is slightly advanced to make up for the incision. At first these operations claimed high success rates in the early 1980s, but it is thought that many patients have since experienced remission of their symptoms after a few months and some women even experience a worsening of their symptoms. Patients with scarring from this operation can benefit from oestrogen therapy.

Anti-oxalate Therapy

Dr Solomons and Dr Melmed have now tried anti-oxalate therapy which involved calcium citrate tablets and a dietary change for more than 100 women with vulval pain, all of whom had abnormal amounts of calcium oxalate in their urine. Of the 25 patients the researchers studied thoroughly, eight experienced complete relief, 12 are able to function normally despite some residual discomfort and five have not responded to this therapy. The research also indicated that women with bladder symptoms suggestive of interstitial cystitis (*see page 42*) have also experienced relief of their bladder symptoms on anti-oxalate therapy.

As well as calcium citrate tablets which dilute the oxalates, the therapy includes an anti-oxalate diet. Complete avoidance of foods high in oxalate is recommended. These foods include spinach, nuts, tea, chocolate, beets, rhubarb, strawberries and wheat bran. Dr Melmed and Dr Solomons stress that women with vulval pain should not attempt to self-medicate. Calcium citrate can be unsafe to use without medical supervision and it can be ineffective if the size and timing of the doses is not based on knowledge of an individual woman's daily oxalate cycle. Seek information from the Vulval Pain Foundation for details (*see page 127*).

As this is a relatively 'new' condition many women with vestibulitis suffer isolation and despair. The most important and effective treatment of all with vulval pain is that your doctor be supportive, accessible, understanding and constantly on the lookout for a specific cause. He or she must be willing to manage the condition with patience and empathy and not succumb to using aggressive therapies easily. For many women, suffering is greatly relieved by the fact that, at last, someone 'believes' them and is taking an interest in their progress.

Complementary Therapy and Pain Management

- Bathing the area with ice bags (*see herpes, page 25*) soothes itching and burning.
- Some women have found relief by taking 1000 mg capsules of evening primrose oil daily for three months. Evening primrose contains GLA which is said to be effective in alleviating hormonal imbalances and this may be why it helps.
- Pure, cold stabilized aloe vera juice can alleviate the burning sensation and can also protect the vulva from irritants.
- Calendula cream is soothing and can help soreness, as can diluted tea tree essential oil and lavender lotions.
- Hypercal cream, a homoeopathic cream for stinging cuts can also help.
- Potassium permanganate, diluted to a very pale pink colour can soothe inflammation.
- Bathing the area with cotton wool soaked with cold, salt water is helpful. Salt baths are also therapeutic as they soothe and heal inflamed mucous membranes.

- Indian tea bags contain tannic acid which is an anaesthetic known to calm burning sensations. Some women get relief by bathing with tea bags in the bath, or by placing a warm tea bag on the area at bedtime.

Prevention

If you can have intercourse, always make sure you are well lubricated, or use a lubricant, as friction on the area can temporarily worsen the symptoms. You may not be able to 'prevent' vestibulitis or vulvodynia in the real sense of the word, but if you experience vulval symptoms, it is important that you do not just assume it is thrush (yeast infection) — get yourself tested for vestibulitis, as the treatment for it is different from that for thrush.

Interstitial Cystitis

Like vulvodynia, this condition has only been recognized by the medical profession fairly recently and countless women have been, or still are, suffering in silence. The symptoms of interstitial cystitis (IC) can be similar to cystitis, but far more intense. They include:

- Burning pain in the abdomen.
- Pressure and discomfort when the bladder is full.
- Chronic urinary frequency (day and night) and relief when voiding.
- Abdominal, urethral, vaginal and vulval pain and/or tenderness.
- Painful sexual intercourse, often intolerable.
- Vestibulitis symptoms, page 33.
- No bacteria in urine test and no relief with antibiotics.

Although this condition was first described in 1830, it has not been recognized by the medical profession until recently, perhaps because it affects 11 times as many women as men. Unlike cystitis which can normally be treated with antibiotics, IC is seen by some as a chronic inflammation of the bladder wall that is not known to be caused by a bacteria, so it does not respond to antibiotics. Some doctors believe it is due to a defect in the blood supply to the bladder and nerves surrounding the pelvic organs. Others say it is due to toxic substances in the urine or defects in the bladder lining. Whatever the cause, the usual urine tests commonly show a 'normal' result, and because of the ignorance in the UK about IC, many women who experience these chronic symptoms are dismissed by doctors as neurotic. Long thought to be a rare disorder of post-menopausal women, interstitial cystitis is now known to be relatively common, and it is being diagnosed more frequently in women in their twenties, thirties and forties.

As a result of increasing awareness in the USA, nearly half a million people have been diagnosed, yet on average, IC patients visit five doctors over the course of two and a half to four years before they get this diagnosis. There is reasonable awareness of the condition amongst British urologists now, but many GPs are still ignorant of it. If you think you are suffering from IC, make sure you are screened for vaginal infections which can have cystitis-like symptoms (such as chlamydia) and if this does not show up anything, insist on being referred to a urologist.

One of the reasons why diagnosis is so difficult is that there is no clear cut test for it and it is usually made by excluding all other possible causes. The only test that can be done involves stretching the bladder with water under general anaesthetic and looking for tiny haemorrhages on the bladder wall. A biopsy of the bladder usually shows non-specific inflammation, but this should be done to rule out bladder cancer.

Treatment

It is important to note that once you develop symptoms of IC, they rarely get any worse and 50 per cent of sufferers can get better without treatment in the first year. After that, the remission rate drops to between 20 and 25 per cent and after five years it is 10 per cent. This remission pattern makes it quite difficult for doctors to assess whether patients are getting better with therapy, or just getting better anyway. As there is no cure at the moment and treatment is mainly geared to the relief of symptoms, ask your doctor to refer you to a urologist to get a definite diagnosis, then together you can consider the following treatments:

- Bladder distension – stretching the bladder by filling it with water under general anaesthetic can alleviate symptoms, but this may only be temporary.
- Anti-depressants such as Elavil appear to have pain-relieving properties (check about side-effects and avoid alcohol).
- Anti-inflammatory agents such as DMSO can be inserted into the bladder intravenously through a catheter.
- Elimiron – a drug which is said to create a protective coating inside the bladder wall.
- TENS – Electrical stimulation is now a routine treatment for a variety of painful conditions, including labour. Patients wear the TENS unit for eight to ten hours a day like a beeper, with electrical stimulation pads on the thighs and lower abdomen. The device acts to block pain impulses by substituting a different electrical impulse. In a study of 35 patients in Sweden, improvement of symptoms was good or excellent in 16 out of 20 patients[5].
- The most dramatic solution is the removal of the bladder which is said to offer complete pain relief, but this is a last resort.

NON-INFECTIOUS CAUSES OF VAGINAL PAIN

Diet

Many IC patients find that eating certain foods can aggravate a chronically inflamed bladder. The Interstitial Cystitis Support Group in Britain (*see appendix for address*) recommend the following modifications which you can try to see if they help you.

Avoid: beer, wine, carbonated beverages, drinks containing artificial sweeteners and tea and coffee. Substitute with decaffeinated beverages and bottled water to see if this has any effect.

Avoid: all fruits except melon (not canteloupe) and pears. Other fruits contain acid and bananas contain byrosine which can also aggravate.

Avoid: spicy foods including all curries, vinegar, tomatoes, all cheeses (except cottage cheese), pâté, chocolate (except white chocolate), corned beef, mayonnaise, nuts (except almonds), onions and fruit yoghurts.

Complementary Therapy

ACUPUNCTURE

Some sufferers of chronic, painful conditions have found relief after a course of acupuncture – studies have shown that 50 to 80 per cent of people find it effective. The Chinese believe that illness is a result of imbalances in the body's internal energies. Acupuncture uses fine needles to re-establish the proper flow of energy by stimulating certain meridians (energy lines) at vital points in the body to increase or decrease the energy flowing to a particular organ. The needles are usually inserted just under your skin and you may feel a slight tingling. You may need six or seven sessions before improvement occurs.

Some IC sufferers have also found relief through hypnotherapy, and have learned, through self-hypnosis, to control their urinary urges.

Prevention

SELF-HELP

Galvanized by her own experience with IC, Vicki Ratner, an orthopaedic surgeon, formed the Interstitial Cystitis Association in America in 1984 and it now has 15,000 members. As a result of its efforts, four million dollars has been awarded for research and the Association has provided a lifeline for isolated sufferers who are interested in making contact with others. Sufferers in the UK now also have a support group to call on (*see appendix for address*).

Sexuality

Naomi McCormick, an Associate Professor of Psychology at New York State University has done a good deal of research on how this condition can cause sexual difficulties[6]. In her study she found that although many women desired sex strongly, they worried that their constant need to go to the toilet would get in the way of romantic feelings. This anxiety was especially felt by single women who felt this to be a real obstacle in establishing relationships. Several techniques for reducing pain have been developed by sex therapists. McCormick describes them as follows:

> *The couple should experiment with coital positions which minimize the possibility of the penis stimulating the base of the bladder. For example, the woman can get on top of the man so as to control the angle of her partner's penis through her own position. Alternatively, the woman can rest on her hands and knees with her partner entering her vagina from behind. Another relatively pain-free position involves the man sitting on the edge of the bed or chair, with the woman sitting on top and the couple rocking so that the penis rests against the cervix rather than the woman's bladder.*

NON-INFECTIOUS CAUSES OF VAGINAL PAIN
Vaginal Dryness

This is one of the most common causes of superficial pain. The vagina is usually kept moist and healthy by your body's delicate hormone balance. Therefore, at certain times in the monthly cycle when there are hormonal changes in the body, some women find their vaginas are uncomfortably dry and often itchy. This feeling is common after periods, as it takes a while for the natural lubrication of the vagina to return. Some oral contraceptive pills that are high in progesterone can also make you feel dry and women who are breast-feeding may have lower oestrogen levels which can lead to dryness. Other women experience vaginal dryness as a symptom of the menopause (*see menopausal atrophic vaginitis, overleaf*). Stress and anxiety also play a part. Stress affects the levels of oestrogen in the blood and it is this that affects your body's ability to turn itself on. If there's a lot on your mind, your libido suffers and it's more difficult to give yourself over to sexual pleasure. In this situation, your vagina can remain dry no matter what is done to arouse you. Anti-fungal treatments for thrush can also be a cause and if you do go ahead and have sex without adequate lubrication, you're more likely to experience abrasions or bruising to the delicate vaginal tissue, which can trigger attacks of thrush or cystitis and also leave you more vulnerable to transmission of STDs.

Treatments
It sounds corny, but the most important thing is to make sure that you indulge in lots of foreplay, to ensure that the vagina is fully aroused before penetration. Also remember that just because you are a bit dry on one night, it does not mean that your sex life is doomed – just try again when you are a bit more relaxed. Alternatively, find a lubricant that makes sex comfortable (*see menopausal atrophic vaginitis*). If you feel a loss of libido is the cause, this can be difficult to overcome on your own.

If you are finding it difficult to get aroused and well-lubricated during sexual contact, and have tried communicating your needs and desires to your partner without success, perhaps it is time to seek qualified help in the form of sex therapy. It can be highly rewarding.

Menopausal Atrophic Vaginitis

Since the menopause, penetrative sex has become virtually impossible for me. It feels very painful and leaves me sore and inflamed. This has left my partner and I with mutual masturbation which is not very satisfactory. I feel anger that there seems to be little research or help for my 'elderly' condition – as if sex does not matter after the menopause. Oestrogen improves it, but I have not continued with this as my mother died of breast cancer and I am monitored as high risk.

ROSALIND, 65

The decrease in a woman's oestrogen level during the menopause can cause the walls of the vagina to lose much of their moisture and elasticity, and the environment of the vagina can also become more alkaline and prone to infection. If not enough lubricating mucus is produced, the vaginal walls can easily become inflamed and intercourse may be painful as the vagina is too dry and the newly tender, thin mucous membranes of the vagina are easily bruised and/or torn.

Atrophic vaginitis can be a big problem with women who have had a healthy sex life and all of a sudden come to experience pain with intercourse. The symptoms commonly experienced are:

- Vaginal dryness and irritation.
- Pain on entry with intercourse.
- Bleeding after intercourse.
- Persistent cystitis or urinary tract infections.

The urinary problems occur because the urethra (the tube which carries the urine out of the body) also experiences the drying out and shrinkage of healthy tissues and is therefore more prone to infection. With lowered hormone levels, some women also find that their orgasmic response changes. Women may take longer to reach orgasm or have less intense ones and this can also have a damaging knock-on effect on the partner's sexual confidence. Some women can also experience painful contractions, like a muscle spasm, with orgasm.

Treatment

The first step is to find a lubricant that may make sex comfortable. Good water-soluble lubricants include Astroglide and KY jelly. You could also try calendula cream, gel or ointment. Some women find oil-based lubricants more effective but remember you cannot use them with latex condoms as they weaken the latex. Oil-based lubricants include Vaseline, coconut oil or the oil from vitamin E or evening primrose oil capsules. Other women recommend Replens, lubricating suppositories which keep the area moist, but they are expensive for long-term use. Senselle is a vaginal lubricant which can be applied sparingly inside the vagina. Both of these can be applied anytime and don't have to interrupt the lovemaking process. Many women have found that Senselle not only makes sex more comfortable, it can also soothe itching and irritation.

If lubricants do not have the required effect, other treatments involving oestrogen supplementation can keep the vaginal lining plump and lubricated. If painful sex is the only significant symptom experienced with the menopause, most gynaecologists would recommend inserting oestrogen cream into the vagina twice or three times weekly.

Some women such as Rosalind (*see page 48*) worry about the cancer risks of long-term oestrogen use. There are currently no studies that specifically link it with an increase in the risk of cancer, but as the jury is still out, it is up to the woman and her doctor to weigh the risks against the benefits.

In her recent book entitled *The Pause*[7], Lonnie Barbach reported on some interesting solutions for women like Rosalind who still feel apprehensive about taking large doses of oestrogen. Vaginal rings give out very low doses of oestrogen and can relieve symptoms in the vaginal area without going through the body's system. Barbach states that in sufficiently low doses, Estrace cream inserted vaginally can be used safely, even by women who have an oestrogen related cancer. In the USA there is a new vaginal ring which emits only five micrograms of an artificial oestrogen, much less than a woman could apply herself. To date, vaginal rings are not yet available in Britain, but will be in the near future.

If painful sex is just one of many other menopausal symptoms you are experiencing, you may be offered hormone replacement therapy (HRT) where you receive daily doses of oestrogen and perhaps progesterone as well, to balance your own body hormone levels. Long-term studies of HRT use show a 50 per cent reduction, or complete elimination of hot flushes and night sweats, and preservation of the healthy condition the genitals. Although it is under constant scrutiny, the data available at this point tends to indicate that the benefits outweigh the risks. There are, however, women who should only take oestrogen under close medical supervision. These include women with breast cancer risk, uterine cancer, high blood pressure, women who smoke or who have had a stroke. Under these circumstances, oestrogen can be taken orally, through a patch, or oestrogen creams can be applied directly to the vagina.

Complementary Therapy

HERBALISM

Calendula cream is particularly soothing for sore, dry skin, as is vitamin E oil. To soothe itching and irritation, try the therapies recommended for vestibulitis (*see page 38*). Lonnie Barbach observed that the herb chasteberry, drunk as a tea three times a day, can revitalize the vaginal tissue and therefore help alleviate painful intercourse, but it generally takes a few months to experience positive results.

AROMATHERAPY

Aromatherapist Robert Tisserand recommends massaging diluted lemongrass oil into the skin, which encourages oestrogen production. Always dilute 5 drops of essential oil in at least 10 ml of a carrier oil.

Lichen Sclerosis

This is a skin condition which effects the vulva and mostly affects post-menopausal women. The symptoms include:

- Itching on the vulval area.
- White raised patches with a dry, thin parchment surface.

The treatment for lichen sclerosis is usually a limited application of a strong cortisone cream such as Dermovate which has been shown to clear it up effectively. Women with this condition and other skin conditions such as eczema and psoriasis, which can affect the vulva, are advised to wash using emollients such as aqueous cream and to use diluted potassium permanganate to calm inflammation. It is important to have lichen sclerosis properly diagnosed and monitored as it has been associated with abnormal pre-cancerous changes on the vulva in some cases.

Vulval Cancer

This is a rare condition which almost always only occurs in older, post-menopausal women. The symptoms include:

- Chronic vulval itching.
- White thickening of the vulval skin.
- A lump, ulcer or warty mass.

Treatment usually involves the surgical removal of the affected area, or laser treatment. If the cancer spreads into the lymph glands or deep in the pelvis, the prognosis is not good, so if you are in the least suspicious, consult a specialist as soon as possible.

Vaginismus

I'd always hating putting things in my vagina and tampons were a definite no-no. When I attempted intercourse it felt like my partner was cutting into me; I almost expected there to be blood, like I was being ripped open and we had to stop.

JANINE, 22

Vaginismus can be mild or severe and occurs when, for psychological reasons, the muscles surrounding the lower third of the vagina go into spasm and tighten automatically, making penetration impossible or extremely painful.

Why Does It Happen?

This is a complex question and the answer depends on individual circumstances. Ways of thinking which can detrimentally affect our ability to take penetration could have their roots in experiences such as growing up to think sex is shameful or that the vagina is a dirty, secret place. It can also be influenced by traumatic events such as rape or sexual abuse or a particularly difficult childbirth experience. Vaginismus can be due to emotional problems and conflicts in your relationship, or a past relationship, or it can be caused by something as simple as a lack of adequate foreplay and arousal.

Vaginismus can also stem from physical infections; women who associate sex with pain physically because of an infection, may also do so psychologically. If you have had a particularly severe bout of thrush (yeast infection) or a long-term problem with vestibulitis, it is easy to see how you might make a strong association between pain and penetration. The anticipation of pain before or during penetration can lead to the muscles going into spasm resulting in vaginismus. If the pain continues even after the local infection has been treated, it is possible that vaginismus is being maintained by psychological conflicts resulting from the physical experience and this needs to be treated psychotherapeutically. But doctors agree that vaginismus is generally a developmental, psychological condition rather than a physical problem.

Treatment

It is important that all possible physical causes be ruled out before you are referred for treatment for vaginismus. I have had letters from many women, particularly vestibulitis sufferers, who have been referred to psychosexual counsellors for vaginismus when in fact their problems were physical not psychological. This misdiagnosis was not only distressing but also pointless because it did not help their problem. If no physical cause can be found, the first stage of overcoming vaginismus is to find the right help. Ask you GP for advice on seeing a sex therapist, psychosexual counsellor or gynaecologist. Many Family Planning Clinics and hospitals employ psychosexual counsellors who specialize in vaginismus. The best way to overcome it is by getting to the root of the problem and talking it through, rather than resorting to drugs or surgery.

A specialist may try to help in the following ways:

- Listen to your anguish and help to establish the root of the problem. A good specialist is treating you as a person, not just your vagina.
- Some doctors feel that it is not just a woman's problem and will want to see your partner as well if appropriate.
- Help you to get beyond your fears with self-examination and the discovery of your own vagina. This will give you confidence that your vagina is not small or abnormal. It might be suggested that you gradually learn to insert your finger into the vagina, and ultimately, small dilators as well to help you feel comfortable about penetration.
- Other therapists may take a more psychoanalytical approach, discussing your background and dealing with conflicts, anger and other emotions that may be being expressed in vaginismus. It is unlikely that these techniques would include the use of dilators.

Complementary Therapy

Some women have found both homoeopathy and hypnotherapy to be useful in treating vaginismus.

Vaginal Examinations

Another unfortunate side-effect of vaginismus is that many women avoid vaginal examinations such as smear tests, since the contractions of the muscles will not allow the speculum into the vagina. Women who find this procedure painful but still possible may benefit from using local anaesthetic creams such as Xylocaine on the vulval area before the examination. You may also like to ensure that you lessen the incidence of vaginal examinations (and the trauma) by having the examination and any necessary treatment at the same time. For example, when my vestibulitis was at its worst, I was offered a cervical examination under general aneaesthetic so that if anything was wrong, treatment could be carried out immediately without having another painful and traumatic examination while I was awake.

It may be difficult to discuss these issues with your doctor, but it is best to be as straightforward as possible in order that you find a solution which satisfies both of you. Most women with vaginismus, however, will be unable to undergo any vaginal examination involving a speculum until the cause of their vaginismus is resolved. It is worth remembering that diagnosis for a number of vaginal problems such as genital herpes, warts, bacterial vaginosis and vulval vestibulitis can usually be diagnosed without a speculum examination.

Childbirth and Episiotomy

After my episiotomy I was still experiencing painful intercourse 15 months later. It reached the point where I nearly had a nervous breakdown. My husband was close to walking out. I felt confused, battered and unwanted.

LOUISE, 32

An episiotomy is a surgical procedure performed during childbirth; to date it is the most frequently performed operation on women in the West, and it is also one of the most controversial. During most births, especially that of the first child, parts of the vagina tear naturally to allow the baby to pass through. An episiotomy is a surgical incision made by the doctor or midwife, through the skin and muscles of the perineum from the vagina towards the anus, to expand the opening through which the baby will pass (*see fig. 5*). It is supposed to be done only when the baby's health is compromised. However, there has been controversy over its routine use to speed up normal birth procedures (in Britain it is performed in 15–30 per cent of deliveries). Some midwives and doctors believe that the clean cut of an episiotomy

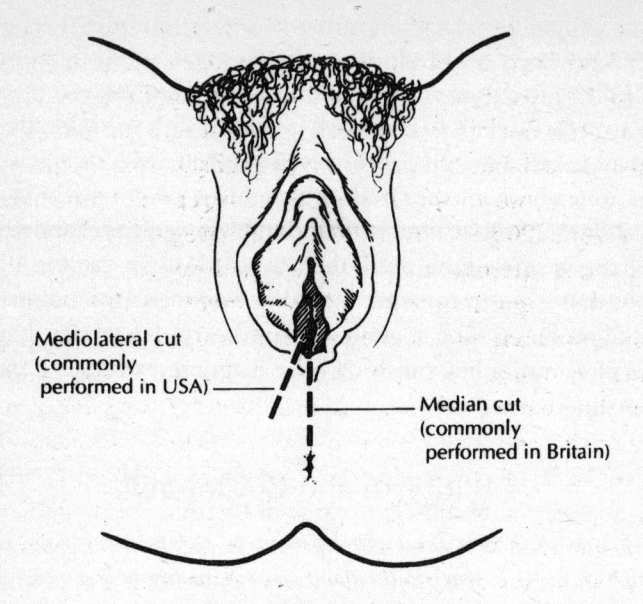

Figure 5: An episiotomy

will heal better than a jagged tear but other research contradicts itself.

Midwifery research fellow Jennifer Sleep conducted a study involving 1000 women at the Royal Berkshire Hospital in 1984. Some 498 women were allocated to a group where episiotomy was withheld and 502 were assigned to a group where liberal use of episiotomy by midwives was allowed. The women allocated to the restricted group suffered more tears and had more intact perineums than those in the liberal group. They also tended to resume intercourse earlier. Sleep concluded:

A policy of using episiotomy to prevent tears does not result in less trauma, improved healing and fewer problems with intercourse ... I would suggest that this rationale be drastically reappraised.

NON-INFECTIOUS CAUSES OF VAGINAL PAIN

About 70 per cent of the women who tear naturally, and all women who have an episiotomy, have some sort of stitching repair to the area after delivery and this can be where the problems start. It is normal to be a bit tender and sore for a few days after giving birth, but extreme soreness after stitching should not persist beyond two to three weeks. Recent reports have shown that as many as 20 per cent of women still have problems such as painful sexual intercourse after three months[8].

Given the magnitude of the problem, there has been surprisingly little research into the best procedures for repair and pain management after childbirth. What is also disturbing is that there is little consensus on the best procedures, with too many professionals carrying on with outdated methods. Concerned about the lack of communication and follow-up about procedures, a research midwife at the Whittington Hospital, Lucy Lewis, completed a research project to audit the clinical standards of midwives and hopefully, to establish how procedures could be improved.

I found an enormous variety in the treatments and advice given to women about relieving the discomfort and pain. Many of these were based on outdated research or folklore, and the midwives had little knowledge of the latest theories on what was best for the woman. This isn't that surprising, as the midwife's care generally ceases at 10 days postnatally and therefore it is not possible for an individual midwife to be aware of the long-term effects of her practice.

What Causes the Problem?

Occasionally soluble stitches, particularly those just inside the vagina, fail to dissolve and do cause irritation. Sometimes the way the stitches have been done may lead to either a vaginal opening that is too tight or to a ridge of unsupported skin at the entrance to the vagina. The scar tissue can also take a long time to heal and becomes painful and itchy. During childbirth, too many women are still dealt with insensitively and are told things like 'you have torn really badly', or 'you are a complete mess down there' just after they have given birth when all they want to do is relax and cuddle their baby. This experience can mean that it takes them a long time to feel 'normal' again, even though the physical cause of the pain has subsided.

Treatment

A midwife or doctor can easily remove any stitches that have failed to dissolve on their own. The ridge of unsupported skin can frequently be relaxed by adequate lubrication and gentle, progressive stretching. Painful scar tissue needs to be able to heal properly. It is best to avoid any trauma (such as intercourse), to the area, as this can slow the healing. You could try gentle intercourse using local anaesthetics such as lignocaine. Some women have found that calendula cream and vitamin E oil help promote healing, but keep in mind that creams should never be used on an open wound. Vitamins E and C taken orally may also help promote the healing process. If the stitches are too tight, or the wound becomes unclean and develops a bacterial infection, the cut is usually made and stitched up again under general anaesthetic.

As mentioned earlier, many of the treatments given by midwives to relieve perineal pain are drawn from complementary therapies and are sometimes not backed up by research, so you may hear of others that are not listed here. The most important thing to do is to keep the area clean and dry using plain, cool (preferably boiled) water on cotton wool pads, or by using small amounts of witch-hazel. Ice-packs are the most common form of relief in the first few days; these can be best applied by putting crushed ice wrapped in muslin onto a sanitary towel which will mould to your shape. Oral painkillers such as Aspirin can also be taken.

Complementary Therapy

AROMATHERAPY

One popular treatment is to apply 2–5 drops of lavender oil to the bath. Lavender has healing and antiseptic properties.

HOMOEOPATHY

A second treatment is to take 30c *arnica* tablets which help bruising.

Prevention

As we have seen, pain can be prevented if you receive the best individual treatment in the first place. A survey in 1993 by the National Childbirth Trust in Britain, showed there were clear differences in the practices used and the pain women experienced[9].

In general terms though, women finishing labour with an intact perineum (no tearing or episiotomy) tended to describe themselves as having 'slight discomfort' postnatally. Mothers with wounds most often said that they had 'definite discomfort' (43 per cent) and mothers who had an episiotomy and tears said they suffered 'pain' (44 per cent).

In the same study, women who had their babies at home were most likely to have an intact perineum, and those who had been told to pant and relax their way through the second stage of labour, rather than push, avoided an episiotomy. Subcutilar suturing is a style of stitching which is more difficult for a midwife to do but is associated with less pain and problems in the future. If possible, request that this style of stitching be done if you require stitches. The materials used are also important. Catgut, which was commonly used until recently, has been associated with more problems than polyglycolic materials such as Dexon and Vicryl. More important than the materials, however, are the skills of the person who carries it out. Until 1985 the task was delegated to medical students but the British Royal College of Midwives' Representatives have campaigned to put a stop to this outrageous practice. Now trained midwives mainly do the repair work, but Lucy Lewis feels that even their training could be dramatically improved.

> *Basically we had one hour training in a classroom practising on a sponge, and then after three supervised jobs we were left to get on with it. Consequently, the skills you develop vary greatly and there is no opportunity for retraining with revised techniques.*

Another practice which is not properly assessed is whether tears actually need stitching at all. Natural healing is usually fine for small, superficial tears but for deeper ones this will usually involve at least a week's bed rest; not all women would be able to do this. What is important is that women should be aware that there are choices and should be involved at all stages of their postnatal care. For this purpose, Lucy wants to see a role for perineal counsellors, similar to breastfeeding counsellors. They would evaluate the practices of midwives and retrain and inform them of the best, updated techniques when necessary. They would also counsel prospective mothers about perineal care before and after the birth, so that each woman can make an informed decision about episiotomy, tearing and stitching. Women should also receive a postnatal leaflet advising them on how to look after their perineums. As Lucy Lewis explains:

> *I think it's important to facilitate the woman's treatment as a partnership. If a woman has a first degree tear which is not very deep I will explain to her that it can be stitched so that it will heal quickly, or left, so that it can heal naturally. The latter option will take a few days' bed rest, so it will all depend on her individual circumstances and whether she is able to do this. The most important thing is communication and I believe that this can prevent a lot of trauma and future problems.*

NON-INFECTIOUS CAUSES OF VAGINAL PAIN

Prevention Guidelines for All Vaginal Irritations and Infections

Avoid any clothing which encourages sweating in the vaginal area, thus providing a warm, moist environment for bacteria to flourish. Always wear cotton underwear instead of nylon, stockings or pop socks instead of tights and avoid tight trousers or jeans, which can rub and bruise the vulva.

Avoid washing underwear in strong biological washing powders. Do not use products such as feminine hygiene wipes — plain water will do. Using talcum powder, bubble bath and deodorizing soaps can all upset the normal, non-pathological bacteria in the vagina. If you want to indulge yourself at bathtime, try natural products such as Dead Sea or Epsom salts, or a few drops of an aromatherapy oil such as sandalwood.

Natural creams can be soothing, sometimes curative and can be used at the first sign of trouble. Propolis cream made from honey, or unprocessed pure honey which is a natural antibiotic can be used for BV, TV and cystitis. Aloe vera gel has anti-fungal properties and some women have found it soothing for thrush (yeast infection) and vestibulitis. Calendula cream can also be soothing if the skin feels very sore and itchy. I have found calendula, tea tree and lavender oil cream soothing for vestibulitis. All of these can be found at good health shops or chemists. It is worth remembering that vulval skin is extremely sensitive and none of the creams mentioned have been subject to clinical trials. Always put a tiny amount on first and if it stings or irritates, do not use it.

After a bowel movement, wipe your bottom from front to back. This gives less opportunity for bacteria from faeces to wipe onto the opening of the vagina and urethra.

Using condoms will prevent transmission of all vaginal infections apart from herpes and genital warts, and barrier methods such as the diaphragm or cap will protect the cervix from infections such as chlamydia.

Lesbians can avoid vaginal infections by taking care not to transfer fluids between vaginas. If sex toys are used for penetrations, ensure that condoms are placed over them beforehand and that they are changed before you share them.

Even if you can use tampons, cotton sanitary towels are still preferable as tampons are usually made from bleached cotton which contains chemicals which could irritate.

Chapter 3
CAUSES OF DEEP INTERNAL PAIN

So far I have looked at the causes of painful sex which are concentrated on the vaginal and vulval areas, but many women also complain of pain in the lower abdominal area. Very often this pain arises because the arousal level before penetration is not high enough to lift the cervix and uterus away from the upper end of the vagina before deep thrusting begins; as a result, the cervix can get bruised. To avoid this happening, ensure you have indulged in lots of foreplay and are fully aroused before penetration. Using a different position can also solve this problem. Try positions where you can control the level of thrusting, either with you on top, or lying side-by-side facing each other. If you are using an IUD or coil for contraception, this can sometimes be the source of pain with deep thrusting and you need to consult a doctor to check that it is correctly placed. Pain experienced either during thrusting or after intercourse can be a warning sign to infections of your reproductive organs and should be investigated as soon as possible. He or she will probably do an internal examination, or if the cause is difficult to locate, a laparoscopy may be necessary. Some stomach conditions such as constipation and irritable bowel syndrome can also cause deep pain during sex, and it is best to avoid penetration when you are having a bad bout of symptoms.

Retroverted Uterus

This happens when the uterus lies with its top tipped back and the cervix juts forwards into the vagina. Around 10 to 15 per cent of women have a naturally retroverted uterus, although sometimes the condition is caused by endometriosis (*see page 75*). In these cases, scar tissue attaches to the uterus and tips it.

A retroverted uterus can cause pain during intercourse because the ovaries are also tipped backward, and pressure may be exerted on them during intercourse. But the body has its own built-in solution; when a woman is fully stimulated sexually, her vagina dilates and elongates, and her uterus withdraws into the abdominal cavity. Intercourse should not feel painful at this point. But if thrusting occurs in the early stages of lovemaking before you are excited, penetration can be uncomfortable. Indulge in plenty of foreplay and take initial penetration slowly, then you should not have any pain.

If you still feel pain with vigorous thrusting as intercourse progresses, experiment with different coital positions, such as both partners lying on their sides or the woman on top, until you find one you are comfortable with. As a last resort, surgery can be performed to correct the uterus but this is not very popular anymore after disappointing results.

Cervical Erosion

This occurs when cells that normally grow on the inner lining of the cervix appear on the outside. Cervical erosion can be caused by an injury during childbirth, long-term use of the pill, or something you were born with which may, or may not cause you problems. Symptoms include:

- Pain or tenderness in the lower abdomen when thrusting occurs and puts pressure on the cervix.
- Bleeding during intercourse.

Treatment

By taking a cervical smear test or pap smear, your doctor will be able to tell whether cervical erosion is the cause of your problem. Treatment can involve the tissue being cauterized, frozen or treated with lasers.

Pelvic Inflammatory Disease

This is an umbrella term for infections or inflammations that have penetrated deep into the reproductive system. It can affect the ovaries, fallopian tubes and uterus and, if left untreated, can cause infertility. The clinical definition of pelvic inflammatory disease (PID) is notoriously inaccurate since it is not just one condition but has many conditions allied to it, and there is little consensus over what is to be included. Many doctors use the term chronic PID when referring to chronic pelvic pain, pelvic adhesions and tubal blockage. I will adhere to American gynaecologist Dr Berger's definition of PID[1] which is the most universal: that PID is an infection which ascends from the vagina and cervix to the fallopian tubes and sometimes their adjoining structures such as the ovaries, and pelvic cavity (*see fig. 6*).

Salpingitis (an infection of the fallopian tubes) is the most common form of PID. Left untreated, it can lead to chronic ill-health and may cause scarring which blocks the fallopian tubes, increasing the risk of ectopic pregnancy and infertility.

However the big issue with PID is getting an accurate diagnosis. This is difficult because it manifests itself in so many different ways and is often badly managed. Jessica's story is sadly typical:

PAINFUL SEX

I got out of bed one morning and I noticed that it hurt when I stood up and put my feet on the floor, and low down in my stomach even the vibrations of walking hurt me. I went to the doctor who pressed my stomach and said I had some kind of womb infection but he didn't give me an internal examination or antibiotics and he sent me to a Family Planning Clinic. They took pap smears and various tests but nothing showed up. This went on for three years. Deep penetrative sex was very painful and would spark off a feverish flare-up. I avoided sex for a year and a half which didn't do any good to my relationship and I felt like I would never be normal again. I was also worried about my fertility and when I finally did get to hospital and they opened me up for a laparoscopy they found that my tubes were so scarred and infected they had to be removed and consequently I am infertile. Why was this allowed to happen? If you've got something around the area of sexuality and there isn't physical evidence then you immediately fall into the category of being hysterical. The doctors believe their swabs before they believe your subjective impressions and it's tragic.

Symptoms

The symptoms of PID have been identified as the following, but they may vary greatly in their intensity. Unfortunately, the level of discomfort does not always indicate the severity of the infection, so if you have two or more of these symptoms, it is important to see a doctor as soon as possible.

- Lower abdominal pain or tenderness. This may be intermittent or constant and may occur during or after intercourse, menstruation or ovulation (midway between periods). Often the pain is only on one side of the abdomen and increases with movement. Sometimes women also have pain with bowel movements or passing urine.
- Fever with a temperature of around 38°C and occasional chills with a normal temperature.

- Lower back pain.
- Fatigue and lethargy.
- Any abnormal vaginal bleeding such as increased menstrual flow, bleeding between periods or after intercourse.
- Unusual vaginal discharge.
- Tingly pain that goes down the tops and inside of legs.

As a way of helping to define what constitutes PID, some doctors have classified the degree of PID by using the following definitions:

Acute PID

This refers to PID where there is a high level of infection. Abscesses (pockets of pus) may form and although this happens infrequently, there is a danger that they may burst, spreading the infection to the lining of the pelvic cavity.

Recurrent PID

Here, episodes of infection are followed by periods of health. Once the vagina, uterus and tubes are damaged by an infection, they may not recover the natural protective mechanisms, which means that many women may have repeated attacks. Another reason may be that the original treatment failed to kill all the infection. Many doctors prescribe antibiotics for suspected PID before they have found out which bacteria is causing the problem. It may also be that a male partner is reinfecting the woman with an organism known to cause PID. It is very important that your partner is screened at a GUM clinic for sexually transmitted diseases. PID is not just a woman's problem (*see overleaf*).

Chronic PID

When PID is inadequately treated, as in Jessica's case, the infection lingers on for long periods, causing discomfort but no acute pain. Some doctors say this discomfort is not due to the infection but to the effects of the damage to the tissues caused by the infection.

Silent (Sub-clinical) PID

Tragically, this is mainly diagnosed retrospectively when women being evaluated for infertility are found to have tubal scarring associated with PID. It is assumed that an infection has been at work without the patient's knowledge. One estimate gives the ratio of three to one for silent to overt PID, making it much more common than overt PID.

What Causes It?

Chlamydia now accounts for the majority of cases of PID, but unfortunately many people with chlamydial infection are not aware of the problems as there are often no symptoms (*see page 18*). Chlamydia affects the cervix at the neck of the womb, and if untreated, may travel into the uterus and fallopian tubes. About 40 per cent of affected women suffer damage to the lining of the uterus and 20 per cent suffer damage to the tubes from chlamydia. Chlamydia can also be spread from the cervix into the uterus by any kind of medical procedure such as an insertion of an inter-uterine device (IUD), or an abortion; the implications are that women should be tested for chlamydia before these procedures are carried out. Men get a common sexually transmitted disease (STD) known as non-specific urethritis (NSU) and non-gonococcal urethritis (NGU), and it is now known that chlamydia is responsible for up to half of these cases. The symptoms are usually a scanty, milky discharge from the penis and discomfort when passing urine. These men may then pass the infection via their sperm to their partners, who often experience no symptoms and it may go on to cause PID. Unfortunately, as NSU and NGU are easily diagnosed and treated with antibiotics, it is still considered a trivial infection by some doctors. As a result, female partners who may be at risk of a serious condition such as PID, are not always traced. However, if the infection is treated at a GUM clinic partners are usually traced.

Gonorrhoea

Gonorrhoea (commonly known as the 'clap') is also a cause of PID. This is a bacteria which affects the warm, wet linings of the genitals in both men and women. It can also live in the mouth and throat. Gonorrhoea is sexually transmitted either through unprotected intercourse (anal or vaginal) or by oral sex. Most women (two-thirds) have no symptoms, but if symptoms do appear they are as follows:

- Unusual vaginal discharge – thin and watery (often yellow).
- Burning sensation when passing water.
- Pain in the abdomen, just below stomach.
- Irritation in the anus.

Over nine in ten men show symptoms of gonorrhoea which include a white or yellow discharge from the urethra or anus. Diagnosis is made by taking swabs from the urethra, cervix, throat or rectum and it is treated with a range of antibiotics. It is encouraging that cases of gonorrhoea are fast declining[2]. In 1993 in the UK they fell from a peak of 60,000 new cases a year in the 1970s, to 11,000 for 1993, which is the lowest since records began in the 1920s.

Other Causes

Often PID is regarded as a purely sexually transmitted disease and this can be misleading since it can also be caused by infections after surgery. Vaginal douching, which is more widely practised in the USA than in Britain[3] has also been identified as a cause because of the risk of either forcing unwanted bacteria up the cervix, or of altering the vagina's natural pH balance, making it more susceptible to unwanted organisms.

Diagnosis and Treatment

This is difficult as there are a number conditions such as pelvic pain syndrome and endometriosis (*see below*) which have similar symptoms. In the first instance therefore, your doctor should do a pelvic exam. Here the doctor inserts two well lubricated and gloved fingers into the vagina while the abdomen is felt with the other hand. The doctor will look for any abnormal pain and thickening typical of PID. A swab of the cervix will be taken to see if any organisms which cause infection such as chlamydia can be detected. Unfortunately, negative tests do not always mean you are clear of PID because the infection can be lodged higher up in the tubes or uterus as in Jessica's case. At this point, your partner should also be checked to see if he or she is harbouring any harmful bacteria.

An ultrasound test may also be performed to get a picture of the pelvic organs and to see whether any abscesses are present. The test involves having gel rubbed on the lower abdomen, then having a transducer passed over the abdomen, emitting and receiving sound waves through to the abdomen. Ultrasound is able to pick up abnormalities in the soft tissues, unlike x-rays. It is a completely painless and harmless procedure. Some doctors may speculatively give you antibiotics to see if the problem clears. These are likely to be from the tetracycline family of antibiotics which are know to be effective against 90 per cent of the organisms which cause PID.

If the response is not dramatic and your swab tests of the vagi-

CAUSES OF DEEP INTERNAL PAIN

na and cervix are still showing negative, request a laparoscopy. It is only possible to take swabs from the uterus, ovaries and tubes during this uncomplicated procedure which is usually performed in a hospital under general anaesthetic. A tube is inserted into a small incision near the belly button, then carbon dioxide is used to inflate the abdomen so that the doctor can have a clear view of the reproductive and pelvic organs. A laparoscope, a special micro-telescope, is then inserted into the abdomen so the doctor can have a look around.

Another tiny incision is made at the pubic hair line and a probe is inserted to gently move organs around so that the doctor can see more clearly. This procedure will usually reveal swollen tubes, ovaries and scar tissues caused by infection, as well as other problems such as endometriosis. You need plenty of rest after a laparoscopy and if you have troublesome PID at the time, you may experience a flare-up after the procedure.

In the USA, doctors are more likely to do a endometrial biopsy which involves taking a small sample of tissue from the endometrium (womb lining). This can be performed without an anaesthetic and it is supposed to be very accurate. Whatever procedure is used, however, if the results show a specific organism to be the cause of your symptoms, you will be prescribed an antibiotic known to be active against that organism. It is vital that you take the whole course of treatment despite the fact that you may be feeling better, otherwise the infection could linger. In cases of acute PID, antibiotics are given intravenously in hospital, for quicker absorption.

The use of strong antibiotics can leave you feeling run down and vulnerable to other conditions such as thrush (yeast infection). If you are prone to this, use an anti-fungal pessary during the antibiotic course. Many women find that eating live yoghurt or taking acidophilus tablets can help protect against thrush (yeast infection). Make sure you help your immune system by eating a balanced, varied diet with plenty of fruit and vegetables.

Get plenty of bed rest and take time off work until your symptoms have cleared. Women with PID need a great deal of emotional support as the recurrent pain and often disbelieving tone of doctors can be very exhausting.

> *I found the psychological pain the most debilitating. I felt I was never going to be well and have a normal sex life and I was infertile. It's amazing that with all this, counselling was never even suggested.*
>
> JESSICA

Complementary Therapy

Jessica found a cure for PID using a combination of orthodox surgery, acupuncture, homoeopathic remedies and fasting therapies and is convinced that the complementary therapies were critical (*see chapter 6 on complementary therapies*). Unfortunately, the damage to her organs was irreparable and her fertility was not restored.

HOMOEOPATHY

Mag sulph is used to help reduce inflammation in the pelvis and *sepia* is suggested for the 'bearing down' sensation common in PID.

HERBALISM

Echinacea taken internally, improves the capability of the immune system and helps to clear up infection. Take in capsules, or as a tea four times a day.

Prevention

Disturbingly, a diagnosis of PID normally follows a long period of silent infection. Regular gynaecological check-ups, including screening for chlamydia, are an effective way of dealing with such infections prior to the development of PID itself. Using condoms will drastically cut down the risks of infections which cause PID.

There are also risks of transferring bacteria through fingering so make sure you and your partner have clean hands beforehand.

Pelvic Congestion

This occurs when the veins in the uterus become inflamed, sometimes almost three times their normal size in diameter. When the veins become enlarged, they cause slow circulation of blood in the pelvic area causing pelvic pain. It is often confused with PID and more than eight out of ten women, complaining of pelvic pain for which no cause can be found through laparoscopy, are found to have this condition. The symptoms include:

- A dull ache in the lower abdomen which gets sharper with standing or exercise and better with rest. It could be more pronounced on one side than the other.
- Painful periods.
- Pain during and after sex, especially after orgasm.
- Irregular vaginal bleeding.

Yet again, because no specific 'infection' shows up with this condition, many women have been labelled as having psychological problems. It is also very commonly confused with PID (*see above*). A study by Professor Beard at St Mary's Hospital Medical School, London, observed the following in a study of women with chronic pelvic pain[4].

> *One of the more striking features of the history of the women with pelvic congestion is the frequency with which pelvic inflammatory disease has been diagnosed in the past, usually for no other reason than the supposition that young women are more likely to have a sexually transmitted disease... The high rate of gynaecological surgery in young women as a result cannot be justified.*

Beard showed that 91 per cent of women complaining of chronic pelvic pain where no other symptoms could be found, had the dilated veins typical of this condition and 60 per cent had suffered severe emotional disturbance as a result.

For Professor Beard, the most useful way to diagnose the problem is by gently compressing the ovaries either on the abdomen, or during a vaginal examination. He asserts that laparoscopy remains an essential part of the investigation of pelvic pain as it is still the only reliable means of excluding endometriosis (*see page 75*). The veins can also be detected by a pelvic venography and by ultrasound scanning. Pelvic venography is an examination carried out during an acute attack of pain to establish what is going on. First a dye is inserted through a vein in the thigh into the pelvic veins so that they show up under x-ray. Then dihydroergotamine, a drug which acts to narrow dilated veins, is introduced; if it succeeds in reducing the pain, the assumed diagnosis of pelvic congestion is seen to be the correct one.

What Causes It?

The condition is thought to be linked to an excess of the female sex hormone oestrogen which is produced by the ovaries. Alternatively it could be that women suffering pelvic congestion are reacting to normal oestrogen levels. Studies have found changes in the uterus and ovaries suggestive of increased concentrations of, or hypersensitivity to oestrogen.

Treatment

Dihydroergotamine which is also used to treat migraine, can be given by injection to narrow the veins. A hormone drug which quells the activity of the ovaries gives some relief. In some cases HRT (*see menopause*) is considered.

Endometriosis

There are days when I want to scream because I just don't know what to do to take away the pain. At times like this you think you will never be 'normal' again. Then there is no relationship; there is only so much of your pain a partner can bear before he is fatigued and bored by it.

JULIE, 24

Endometriosis is usually found in women between the ages of 25–45 and can cause painful periods, painful intercourse and sometimes leads to infertility. In Britain, the Endometriosis Society estimates that it affects one in ten women. Again, it is a condition which is too often badly diagnosed and treated, and many women have had unnecessary hysterectomies in an attempt to cure it. In a survey of 2000 women with endometriosis, conducted by the Society in 1993, it found that nearly a quarter of the women suffered for 10 years or more before they were properly diagnosed. Of the women who were given hysterectomies, 39 per cent still had pain every day[5].

Symptoms

The symptoms vary enormously and are very wide-ranging. The severity of pain depends on where the endometriosis is sited and does not necessarily relate to the extent of the condition. In many women endometriosis is asymptomatic and may resolve itself spontaneously. It is only a problem when the stray tissues cause pain and internal damage. Symptoms may include:

- Pelvic pain – especially severe period pain which starts at the onset of menstruation and continues throughout the bleeding. You may also experience pain at ovulation, in the middle of your cycle.
- Pain on intercourse.

- Infertility (in approximately 40 per cent of cases).
- Painful urination.
- Painful bowel movements.
- Back pain.
- Swollen, bloated abdomen.

What Causes It?

Endometriosis is a condition which occurs when tissue normally found in the lining of the womb (the endometrium), migrates to other parts of the pelvic cavity and establishes itself there as 'stray' patches of tissue. This stray tissue usually implants itself on the outside of the uterus and fallopian tubes, the ovaries or the bladder and the bowel. Each month, these patches of tissue respond to the fluctuation of female hormones brought on by menstruation, by engorging with blood and then bleeding. Because there is nowhere for the blood to go, it collects and forms painful scar tissue. This causes cramps and pain, symptoms sometimes severe enough for an otherwise healthy woman to become bedridden. Inflammation and scar tissue then form around the patches, with each cycle involving more endometriosis growth and bleeding. Over time, the constant build-up of scar tissue at different sites can lead to adhesions on organs, causing the organs which would normally slide gently against one another to become almost 'glued together'. Sometimes the adhesions form large cysts which cause havoc with ovulation and hormone balance (*see fig. 6*).

Why Does It Happen?

The exact cause is still unclear, however 'retrograde menstruation' which occurs when every woman menstruates may play a part. During menstruation the womb lining is shed down into the vagina, but a small amount of the lining falls back along the fallopian tubes into the pelvic cavity where it usually forms tiny implants and disappears. In around 10 per cent of women, the

CAUSES OF DEEP INTERNAL PAIN

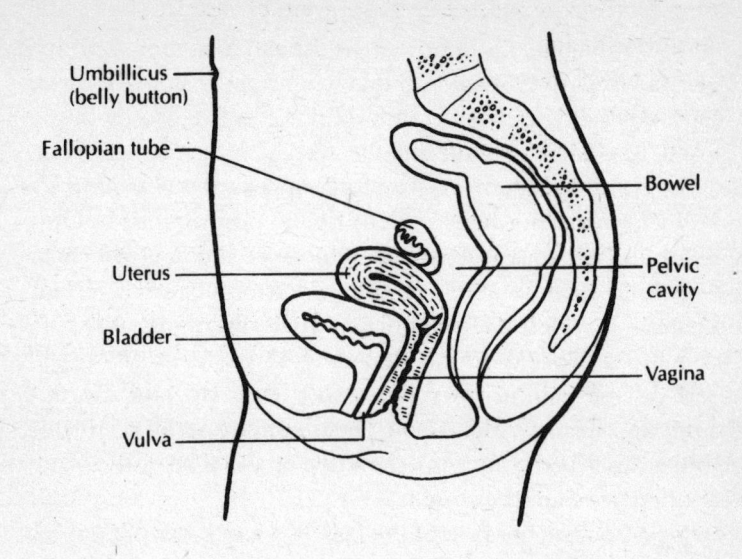

Figure 6: The usual sites of endometriosis

implants grow larger, responding to female hormones and cause damage. Other theories suggest that endometrial tissue is carried through the body's lymphatic system. Genetic factors may also be an influence as one study showed that seven per cent of women with endometriosis had a relative with the condition. There has been considerable interest in the more recent idea that women with endometriosis have some sort of immune deficiency which allows the patches to develop. Some scientists believe that the development of endometriosis may be linked to the increased number of menstruations women now have over a lifetime, because women can control their fertility. Unfortunately, this thesis has led to women being led to feel that it is their fault if they have endometriosis – it is the 'career woman's (childless) disease'. This sort of labelling by the medical profession does nothing to help the condition and is completely unacceptable.

How Is It Diagnosed?

An accurate diagnosis is important as the inflammation and scar tissue can build up every month that it is left untreated. Research by the Endometriosis Society showed that it is still grossly misdiagnosed. The Society found that the average time it took to diagnose the condition after the symptoms appeared was around six and a half years. This delay is partly due to misdiagnosis but it is also due in part to a widespread reluctance among women to consult their doctors about symptoms such as painful periods and painful sex. Despite its significance in terms of diagnosis, the Endometriosis Society found that only 42 per cent of women openly discuss painful intercourse with their doctors. Do not become another statistic; if you persistently experience this or the other described symptoms, see a doctor and if he or she is not sympathetic, see another one.

Delays also arise because of the lack of a quick, simple test for endometriosis. A doctor can check the position of the uterus and find certain signs suggestive of endometriosis; it is, for example, more common in women with retroverted uteruses (*see page 64*). The only way to diagnose it with any certainty is by laparoscopy (*see PID*) — a minor operation in which a small telescope is inserted through an incision in the abdomen which enables the doctor to look for signs such as blisters or cysts. Research at John Radcliffe Hospital, Oxford is currently looking to develop less invasive tests for diagnosing the condition. Although not yet ready for patients, they have developed a blood test which shows certain antibodies in the blood which are markers for the presence of endometriotic tissue.

Treatments

Endometriosis relies on the chemicals involved in the menstrual cycle to trigger and encourage its development. Therefore, one way to clear it, is to stop menstruation for about six months to allow healing to take place. Pregnancy is seen as the best way to do this as during pregnancy the implants rapidly shrink, and in some cases, may not return after childbirth. A recent study in Oxford confirmed that pregnancy also can protect against the disease. But becoming pregnant is not a practical solution for everyone. Firstly, around 40 per cent of women with endometriosis have infertility problems and pregnancy is not an option. Also it may not be practical or desirable for the individual woman, especially lesbian and single women, to conceive and have a child. They should not be made to feel that they are preventing a 'cure' because of this.

Medical hormone treatments are another option as they emulate the pregnant or menopausal state. The combined oral contraceptive pill is often used for a period of six to 18 months. Other forms of hormone therapy include Danazol (Danol), a synthetic derivative of the male hormone testosterone. It acts by discouraging oestrogen production in the body and without active oestrogen, most implants will shrink and die away. Danazol can only help to resolve the actual patches of tissue found in mild and moderate cases of endometriosis and cannot heal the scar tissue or adhesions found in more severe cases. It can also have unpleasant side-effects such as thickening of facial and body hair, skin problems, muscle cramps and joint pains. To allay any anxiety discuss these side-effects fully with your doctor before undertaking hormone therapies. A good exercise workout three times a week is said to lessen these side-effects.

A more recent drug, Gestrinone has similar effects to Danazol. One study, using the drugs on two separate groups, showed that after six months, the symptoms in both the treatment groups had improved, but the group taking Gestrinone found it easier to take and had fewer side-effects[6]. Naferlin is a temporary menopause-inducing drug and has also been associated with fewer side-effects than Danazol. In a trial of 82 patients with symptoms including painful periods, painful intercourse and pelvic pain, as many as 94 per cent improved with Naferlin. It is taken as a nasal spray, usually sprayed twice daily between days two and four of the menstrual cycle[7].

For some women, hormone therapy is not the whole answer and its relief may only be temporary. In these cases surgery is often considered, depending on the degree of symptoms, the extent of the damage and the woman's desire for children. Minimally invasive surgery, often involving laser treatment is used to 'burn off' the endometriosis implants. The most extreme form of surgery is hysterectomy, the removal of both ovaries, but this is not always completely effective and can cause menopausal symptoms. Some experts now believe that between 70 and 90 per cent of women with chronic abdominal pain from endometriosis can be helped by one of these therapies, but extensive research into the causes and more palatable treatments still needs to be done. Scientists are currently investigating how endometriotic tissue grows and invades other tissues. Research is also going on in the UK regarding a coil which releases hormones into the system with few side-effects. Initial trials on endometriosis patients showed success at relieving pain.

Complementary Therapy

Supplements to boost the immune system and regulate hormone balance have proved very helpful to many women with endometriosis. The B vitamins, particularly B6 have been popular for counteracting feelings of lethargy and depression. They are also thought to help regulate oestrogen balances. Evening Primrose Oil has an effect on pain and inflammation and appears to reduce the side-effects of hormone therapy. Selium ACE (vitamins A, C and E) can strengthen the immune system and vitamin E prevents scar tissue from thickening.

Sex

Only participate in intercourse if you feel comfortable. It may be easier if you are on top of your partner, as you can control the depth of penetration more easily. Hormonal treatment may lead to a dry vagina, so do not be embarrassed about using lubricants such as KY jelly.

After-effects of Hysterectomy

Many women approach the idea of a hysterectomy with a great deal of anxiety because its consequences are dramatic and irreversible. In reality, hysterectomy has advantages and disadvantages. The reason you are having the operation, how informed you are about the procedure and its effects, your feelings about fertility and the stability of your relationship will all have an effect on your experience of hysterectomy.

What Is It?

The most common operation performed today is a 'total hysterectomy', meaning the removal of the uterine body plus the cervix. In pre-menopausal women the ovaries are conserved to avoid premature menopause, but in post-menopausal women, they will often be removed. In a partial hysterectomy, only the body or upper part of the uterus is removed and the cervix is left in place (*see fig. 7*). Any women who is told she needs a hysterectomy for any reason should get a second opinion, especially in America where 33 per cent of women have had one by the age of 65, a figure generally considered to be unreasonably high. The most common condition leading to hysterectomy is cancer of the uterus, ovaries or Fallopian tubes, uncontrollable uterine bleeding, fibroid tumours and endometriosis (*see above*). For older women, hysterectomy is sometimes advocated for relatively mild problems on the basis that after child-bearing, the uterus becomes a relatively 'useless' and potentially cancerous organ and is best removed. One wonders if the same male gynaecologists would similarly advocate the removal of the prostate in men, an operation which can easily be compared to a hysteretomy.

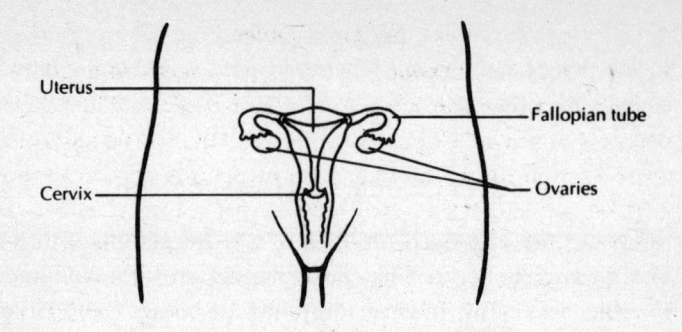

Figure 7: Intact (before hysterectomy)

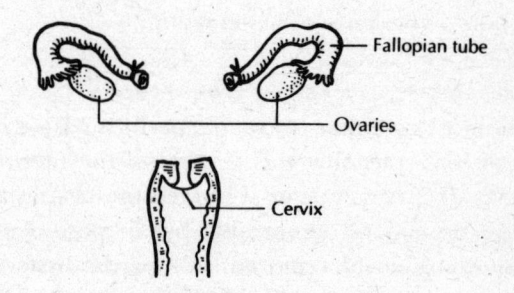

Subtotal hysterectomy (only uterus removed)

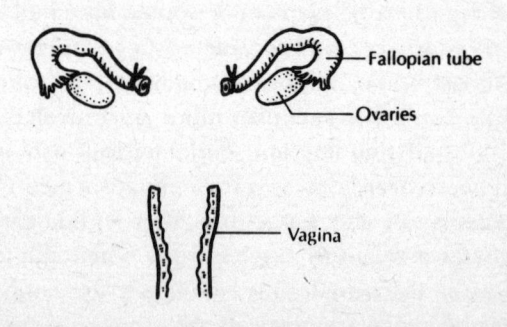

Total hysterectomy (uterus and cervix removed)

Sexual Problems

Sexual problems following hysterectomy occur in a minority of women, but they can have a debilitating effect. The loss of the uterus (known in China as 'little heart') may negatively affect some women for whom uterine contractions were an important part of orgasm. It can also have a psychological effect, as the removal of the uterus symbolizes the end of a woman's fertility and that aspect of her womanhood which may have contributed to her sexual identity. Women with these feelings may experience lowered self-esteem and depression which can cause sexual problems. In addition, both the woman and her partner may fear that intercourse could harm the wound in some way. Decreased hormone levels due to removal of the ovaries can result in shrinking vaginal tissues and other menopausal symptoms. If the cervix is removed, shortening of the vagina may make intercourse difficult until the vaginal tissues have been dilated or stretched again.

Treatment

If you are experiencing any of these problems after a hysterectomy go back to the doctor; he or she should be able to advise on helpful measures. Sometimes some ovarian residue is left behind after a hysterectomy causing painful intercourse; this can be removed by further surgery.

Prevention

Obviously, whether the operation and it effects can be prevented at all will depend on the reasons why a hysterectomy is prescribed in the first place. A woman with advanced uterine cancer will have completely different issues to evaluate than a woman with endometriosis where the use of hysterectomy is more controversial. However, every woman has a right to have any possible effects on her sexuality explained to her in a non-judgmental way before she undergoes the operation. Women who have made the decision at their own pace are more likely to recover quickly and have fewer sexual and emotional problems after surgery. You need to think about what effect not having all of your reproductive organs will have on your self-image. You may also need to consider the reaction of others after you have had a hysterectomy and what effect that will have on your relationships with them. Many women have expressed feelings of anger about the sense of betrayal and isolation they felt as a result of their treatment, principally because they were not fully informed about the procedure or its effect.

Hysterectomy As a Cure For Painful Intercourse

A recent study in New Zealand of sexuality and hysterectomy[8] emphasized the importance of information prior to surgery, indicating that when this occurs, the sexual satisfaction of the woman is not usually detrimentally affected. This group of women were provided with an informational booklet by their doctor before their hysterectomies and were questioned about their sexual satisfaction one year later. Forty two per cent reported improvement in their sexual lives following hysterectomy and 52 per cent said there was no change. The few women who experienced negative sexual effects were usually cases where surgery had affected the vagina.

A more recent British study conducted with 400 women who were interviewed a month before and a year after a total hysterectomy, showed that 83 per cent of the women who had suffered from deep pain during intercourse experienced relief after the operation[9].

Chapter 4
THE EMOTIONAL EFFECTS OF PAINFUL SEX

A woman's identity, her perception of herself as a woman, her femininity and her self-confidence are closely bound up with her body image and her sexuality. Sexuality is not just about sex – it is about who we think we are, how we see ourselves, how we think others see us and how we express ourselves in our intimate relationships. Painful sex attacks the core of many women's perception of these things, and although the physical causes or manifestations may vary from person to person, the emotional problems are often very similar. It is amazing that pain in such a small area of the body can have such a profound effect on the whole of your being. Issues of sexuality and illness, particularly in the area of gynaecological illness, are still grossly misunderstood and under-researched, which compounds the sufferers' isolation, and may impede the healing process.

In this chapter I will try to address this yawning gap and acknowledge the problems that can occur. The emotional responses you experience as an individual will depend on your sexual orientation, past sexual experiences, cultural background and expectations, and the quality of the relationship you are in. I will therefore not attempt to prescribe miracle cures here, as finding something that will work to heal you and make you feel happier will depend on taking into account all the above factors.

You may find that you deal with these problems by using coping methods already established in your relationship, or by the love and care of friends, relatives and health-care professionals. I hope that I can help you by confirming that the anguish you may be suffering is real and understandable, and give you the courage to seek professional help in the form of sex therapy, counselling or psychotherapy if appropriate. Women are conditioned to be good, compliant patients – especially in areas where sexuality is concerned, it is tempting to continue suffering in silence. You deserve better!

Silent Anguish

In the course of my research I have interviewed many women with a wide variety of problems in this area, and the same feelings are expressed again and again. They include feeling:

- Guilt: because as women we are supposed to be sexually available and fertile.
- Anger: why me and why does no one help me or believe me?
- Mutilated: feeling freakish as if you were carrying an invisible disability or shameful secret.
- Inadequate: feelings of poor self-esteem. If I can not be sexual who is going to want me; and if I can not be sexual, then can I be any good at anything?
- Self-blame: feelings of being punished for being sexual. Is this illness my fault? Was I too 'promiscuous'?
- Isolated: firstly, because you feel you are the only person this is happening to, and secondly, because these conditions affect what society sees as taboo areas – vaginas and reproductive organs – it may be difficult to share your problem.

THE EMOTIONAL EFFECTS OF PAINFUL SEX

- Anxiety: will it ever go away? Will I ever be normal? Will I find the right help and treatment?
- Depressed: chronic pain and illness can sap your energy and spirits, and can lead to depression.

All this amounts to a hefty emotional burden if it was being carried by a physically healthy woman, let alone a woman suffering the exhaustion and depression associated with chronic pain. These feelings also occur because Western society generally, is unable to speak honestly about sex. You do not have to be a woman with problems in this area to see that the essence of sex, an act of love between two people, is often lost in the deluge of advertising, magazine articles and films obsessed with performance – how many times a night, how many times a week, technique and orgasm frequency. Sex is rarely spoken about except in those terms, therefore if you have a problem you can feel totally alone.

Particularly painful for heterosexual women is that the legitimacy of marriage is tied up with penetration. This is demonstrated by the fact that a marriage can be legally annulled if consummation has not taken place. This fact alone may make you feel very vulnerable if you feel unable to have penetrative sex. So long as we attach shame to sexual problems, or believe them to be rare or self-inflicted there will be no space for problems to be discussed. Thankfully, HIV has brought sexual health into the forefront and hopefully it will highlight the need for honest, frank approaches to sex and the prevention of problems.

Taking the Sting Out of the Doctor's Words

For many women, significant emotional disturbance is caused by the constant demoralizing battle with doctors that they have had to endure in order to find a diagnosis, or treatment for their condition. As Susan Heitler[1], a clinical psychologist, explains:

Reading medical detective stories may be fun, but having a medical problem that has not yet been labelled or understood is not. Doctors' emotional reactions to complaints they do not understand or know how to treat vary. Some sincerely and apologetically acknowledge their inability to help. Others blame the patient when attempts to cure prove useless or even detrimental.

The following cases show this clearly.

I cannot forget the desolation of returning home from my numerous visits to the doctor's feeling no further forward in finding out what was wrong with me. How alone I felt.

TRACEY, 30, SUFFERS FROM VESTIBULITIS.

Despite my pleas, nobody showed any interest in how I was feeling or what was wrong with me. I became scared of being obsessed with the condition and stopped going to doctors even though the pain, or fear of pain was ruining my life.

MICHELE, 24, SUFFERS FROM RECURRENT THRUSH (YEAST INFECTION).

It took me two and half years to be diagnosed (with vestibulitis). My doctor showed no interest whatsoever, but did eventually refer me to a clinic where all the tests were negative. I then saw a hospital gynaecologist who told me I must be 'doing it wrong' and 'had I had sex before?' This was in front of a number of male medical students.

DIANE, 27

THE EMOTIONAL EFFECTS OF PAINFUL SEX

Careless words from your doctor can also make you feel worse about your condition and can sometimes impede your treatment.

I couldn't believe it when I confidently told the doctor that my partner was very understanding about our lack of penetrative sex. He cynically replied 'oh yes, they all say that and I find it very peculiar'. I was feeling so vulnerable at the time, I just wanted to punch him.

TRACEY

In her book on vaginismus, Linda Valins[2] acknowledges that a doctor's words or actions can actually cause the condition. Traumatic pelvic examinations or cervical smears can have lasting effects, as can words such as 'you are a bit small down there', 'you will have a lot of trouble when you get married ...'. Indeed, one women doctor recently said to me *when I was already traumatized by vestibulitis*, 'you are very small down there, I'd be surprised if sex will ever be pain-free.' The fact that doctors almost always assume every woman is sexually active and bypass vaginismus as a diagnosis, or diagnose it in such an insensitive way – 'it's all in your head (your own fault)' or 'you are frigid' – that it can damage the chances of successful treatment.

Women with vaginismus can go through a lot of painful and intrusive investigations by doctors trying to find the cause of their pain and this confirms to them that there is something physically wrong. Then to be told 'we have found nothing, it's all in the mind' leaves women with a terrible feeling of resentment and anger. They are then very difficult for a psychosexual counsellor to treat, because they come with all this feeling of rejection and rage which is hard to work through to find the real cause of their pain.

DR HEATHER MONTFORD, PSYCHOSEXUAL COUNSELLOR

Linda Valins emphasizes that this type of vaginismus can be avoided by pointing out to doctors and nurses, ideally during training, that vaginismus can actually be induced by a rough physical examination or an insensitive approach. She also suggests that when medical staff are conducting a vaginal examination the use of the word 'small' should be avoided and so should any comment that would imply that the shape or look of the vagina is in anyway abnormal unless, of course, this is due to infection.

I would echo the view that medical professionals need to learn counselling and listening skills. An area such as this needs to be treated with the utmost sensitivity and doctors should take it upon themselves to keep abreast of the up-to-the-minute practices.

Susan Heitler[3], explains how her patient Linda, a sufferer of vulval pain, learned how to deal with doctor's comments.

Blaming comments made to Linda included accusations of not using medication properly or using it as a way to avoid sex with her husband. Linda found it helpful to talk openly about such comments with family, friends and therapist. They echoed the view that the doctor's accusatory words came from a sense of helplessness. The problem was her pain, not something wrong with her as a person.

Becoming a patient can be very stressful. A normally responsible woman, who may be used to feeling in control of other parts of her life, surrenders her autonomy and becomes relatively powerless in the hands of powerful professionals. If a woman is suffering from a gynaecological problem, she needs, more than ever to have an open and mutually understanding relationship between her and her doctor. The answer is to shop around until you find a doctor who is sympathetic. No matter how much time or emotional energy it takes, it will be worth it in the end to find someone who is capable of giving you the right diagnosis, discuss treatment options if there are any and truthfully outline the possibility of side-effects. Remember that there may be no magical cure for your condition but it is important to find a sympathetic ear.

Sexual Problems as a Result of Painful Sex

Painful intercourse can lead to many unhealthy sexual responses. As this area is currently very under-researched and under-recognized, many women and their partners do not get the support they need to deal with the problems that arise. Too often, the physical symptoms are treated with virtually no acknowledgement of the emotional disturbance that goes with it.

Sexual Avoidance

It is not uncommon for a woman who finds sexual contact painful to reject all of her partner's sexual advances as a protective measure, out of fear of being hurt and also as a way of seeing herself as non-sexual, incapable of giving or receiving pleasure. Because of her pain, she is not *allowed* to be sexual, therefore does not want to participate in any activity which reminds her of her inadequacy, nor does she want to be reminded of, or have to satisfy, her partner's sexual needs. Not surprisingly, this contributes to anger and disharmony in an intimate relationship, and can prohibit a single woman from feeling confident about establishing a new relationship which may lead to sexual relations.

It also may be the case that the partner interprets a few rejections, when things genuinely are too painful, as a sign that penetration can never be attempted and then the partner worries about inflicting hurt. They will therefore be reluctant to initiate sex, even though the woman may want her partner to do so.

Sacrificing Your Needs

The opposite response may also occur. Under pressure a woman may feel the need to have sex even when it hurts. She may be doing this for herself – to try and confirm her 'normality' — or she may be doing it for her partner – to give him pleasure and to be seen to not be 'denying' him anything. However, this may be very destructive behaviour, as it could increase the woman's repugnance towards sex – she is not expressing herself, but burying her own sexuality and missing the opportunity to find alternatives that could give her pleasure. It may also increase her depression and the sense of isolation.

The vast majority of women who suffer with this problem have reported that their partners are very sensitive to their feelings and health status, and in some cases their sex lives have improved as the emphasis is taken away from penetration in favour of experimenting with other more satisfying sexual practices. However, many women feel guilty about interfering with their partner's pleasure. I have been living with my partner for six years and still feel uneasy about making a marriage commitment because I feel as if I would be 'trapping' him into a compromised sex life for the foreseeable future. I have now come to see that this is an irrational response, but an understandable one.

Secondary Vaginismus

In some cases painful intercourse due to an infection can result in vaginismus which then makes intercourse more painful or impossible. Even when the original source of the pain is removed, the fear of pain and presence of anxiety can inhibit arousal, which results in a lack of vaginal lubrication and causes further difficulty and pain. The muscles at the front part of the

THE EMOTIONAL EFFECTS OF PAINFUL SEX

vagina may involuntarily go into spasm as a defence making penetration difficult. Known as secondary vaginismus (*see vaginismus*), this condition could be prevented if women were given the space to discuss how their condition affects their sexuality while they are experiencing the physical symptoms. As Doctor Montford explains:

> *I have seen a number of women whose vaginismus appears to have started when they had persistent thrush (yeast infection) and that they began to feel themselves as dirty, unacceptable and damaged as a result. Maybe some discussion of the psychological aspects of the condition at the time with the doctor might have avoided that. If a woman feels that she is likely to develop sexual problems and needs help to cope she should ask for it as this way further sexual problems can be prevented.*

It is also useful, if possible, to familiarize yourself with the workings of the vaginal muscles so that you can try to be aware of relaxing and tensing them. Tightening these muscles may have been an exercise that you used in the past to enhance intercourse. Insert a well-lubricated, clean, nail-clipped finger into the vaginal entrance. Now clench the area as if you were stopping yourself from passing urine, then relax. The muscles you have just used are the vaginal muscles. Before you attempt intercourse, you can try this technique to ensure that you are fully relaxed.

Loss of Libido and Sexual Problems

If your sexuality has been associated with pain and your sex life is a cause of emotional conflict, it is not surprising if your libido suffers. Libido is also linked with body image, how you see yourself and how you think others see you. When you experience painful intercourse your body image can become extremely low

– you may see your body as a source of punishment and pain rather than pleasure. I put on over 9.5 kg (25 pounds) in weight when my vestibulitis was at its worst and I now see this not only as a symptom of my depression, but also a way of building some sort of protective shield around my sexuality and desirability.

Libido problems for women can manifest themselves in a number of ways, ranging from arousal problems such as lack of lubrication, to complete lack of interest. It is a good idea to accept that arousal may take a little longer for a woman who experiences painful sex. You may have to compensate by indulging in more foreplay and perhaps using a vaginal lubricant. If the problem goes deeper than this, Dr Montford suggests the following:

> *It would be good for the woman to acknowledge loss of libido with someone such as therapist or counsellor who can give them an insight into the reason for their loss of libido. It may be because they no longer feel a sexual person, it may be because of an unconscious anger and resentment against all men who they may see as being the ones who give disease. It could be connected to something further back in the woman's past. Once the causes are discovered, the problem can be solved.*

Experiment With Pleasure

Many women feel that their sexual arousal is impaired because even when they are free of pain, they feel anxious that the pain might return and ruin their experience. But a study by Whipple and Komisaruk, authors of the now-famous book on female orgasm entitled *The G-Spot*, reported that vaginal stimulation can actually increase the threshold to pain. It is highly feasible then, that on some occasions, for some women, the involvement in sexual stimulation diminishes uncomfortable vaginal sensations.

Indeed one vestibulitis patient reported that the thing that gave her most relief from her symptoms was receiving oral sex from her partner.

Simple measures can be taken to ensure the maintenance of intimacy. If your problem is worse in the evening, try to change your sexual habits to take this into account and initiate contact in the morning. Giving and receiving oral sex, which involves licking and sucking each other's genitals, is a normal and pleasurable part of lovemaking and is widely practised around the world. It can involve as much, if not more, touching and caressing as intercourse.

Stop Deprivation – Give Yourself Pleasure

Take time to get back in tune with your body by having a warm bath with soft music in the background, or indulging yourself with a massage. Find ways to treat yourself sensually and if you indulged in masturbation before your condition developed, there is no reason why this should suddenly stop. You may find new ways to experience this aspect of your sexuality more fully. It is also a convenient way of getting sexual satisfaction, as you are able to pick a time when you are relatively free of pain, and you have total control over the areas of stimulation.

Lesbian women often adapt to sexual adjustment more easily than heterosexual women because they already engage in a variety of sensual experiences and do not place as much emphasis on penetration and intercourse. Generally, with all the conditions mentioned in the book, heterosexual women will find sexual intercourse much easier if the woman takes charge of inserting the penis into the vagina. This can be done most successfully with the woman on top or with both partners lying side-to-side. That way, the woman can control the thrusting and if the penis needs to be withdrawn quickly, it is easy to do. Some sort of distraction from the pain during sexual activities can also help you to overcome it and add some excitement. Many women have indicated that they have done this successfully by maintaining powerful sexual fantasies, dressing up, using sex toys and other stimulations like erotic videos which helped them to achieve normal levels of arousal and allowed them to explore their sexuality in a variety of ways. Mutual massage, mutual masturbation, enjoying each other's bodies, sharing fantasies and mutual bathing are ways in which you can enjoy yourself with your partner when intercourse is difficult.

Your Partner

It would be naive to assume that the difficulties you experience with sex would not in some way affect your partner. Intimacy involves closeness, sharing and trust which is mutual give and take. The people who care about you and have lived this experience with you, feel some of your pain, if only at an emotional level. Their hurt, frustration, concern and fear are just as real as yours.

The emotions a male partner experiences may be multiple and conflicting. On the one hand, he may feel guilty: he may have passed on an infection to you which has caused your distress; or he desires to penetrate you which he knows will hurt you. On the other hand, he can feel deprived, rejected and cheated, and vulnerable to the stereotypical view that women do not like sex and will do anything to avoid it. If these feelings are left unconfronted he is also at risk of developing sexual aversion and erection problems, such as impotence. For both male and female partners, helping them to develop tolerance and acceptance is the best way to avoid these problems. You can do this either by communicating your feelings yourself, or it may be worth visiting a doctor together so that the doctor can fully explain your condition and its implications. Hopefully this will help your partner feel part of the treatment process and obliged to be understanding. Talk as much as possible about your needs and expectations. For example, if you have to stop a sexual encounter because of pain make sure he or she interprets the message as 'ouch, let's do *this* instead', rather than he or she is clumsy and doing something wrong. Ask questions about how you can best please each other. There are many ways in which you can still give and receive pleasure, even if it's a deep passionate kiss.

Seeking Help

If you find that it is hard to deal with the emotional effects of painful sex on your own, or you wish to receive some guidance, consulting a sex therapist, counsellor or psychotherapist can be useful. Indeed some gynaecologists have argued that women who face any kind of physical problem in this area should receive therapeutic support. Any type of sex therapy, psychotherapy or counselling is not something that is done to you, it is something that you participate in yourself and you have to be prepared for this. It does not mean that you are ill and have to be treated; it is a chance to let your voice be heard. Before your first visit, it may be useful to make a list of feelings that concern you. Traditional sex therapy, as pioneered by Masters and Johnson, often involves assessing the problems you are experiencing, which is then followed by homework which the couple, or individuals do at home. Often agreements will be negotiated on how frequently the couple have intercourse, if appropriate, or which type of activities will be engaged in. It is also a time to learn about normal physical responses, foreplay techniques, intercourse positions and how to communicate needs, feelings and wishes.

This form of therapy has been criticized as too 'couple centred', neglecting the needs of single people, and too focused on the immediate problem, rather than the background to it.

Christine Baker, a clinical psychologist in Jersey who specializes in the treatment of male and female sexual problems, believes that therapy should be more aware of the individual's culture and sexuality and the psychological and physical factors which contribute to the problem. She recommends what is known as a 'cognitive behavioural' approach.

It is the individual's attitude to their problem which is considered instrumental and consequently the goal of therapy would be to focus on adjusting the faulty or unrealistic assumptions the person has about what constitutes sexual fulfilment.

For example, for a woman who is experiencing painful intercourse, seeing herself as a 'failure' in that sense can be a self-fulfilling prophecy which increases feelings of hopelessness and inadequacy. Christine would hope to tackle this by challenging the assumption of 'failure' helping the woman to take on a more positive role. It may help to encourage you and your partner to focus on and derive pleasure from a number of different parts of the body and to see this as a rewarding experience in itself, not as a preliminary to the real point such as penetration or orgasm.

Self-esteem

The pain and anguish of these conditions can cause your self-esteem to plummet. Many of the women I interviewed said that they had become much more withdrawn and introverted since their conditions and were often unable to join in social activities or communicate fully with their friends. Maria Hull, a psychotherapist writing in the *Vulval Pain Newsletter*, has a number of recommendations.

Allow yourself to be nurtured by others. You need it and you deserve it. A physical illness is not a character flaw so do not punish yourself by keeping others at a distance. After a while, even the most loving and dedicated friend or family member may back off if they have their heads nipped off, so to speak, too many times. Try not to punish them for being well.

Don't suffer in silence. Tell some significant people in your life how you feel, both physically and emotionally. People who care about you are interested in what you are going through. You do not really 'spare' them by keeping it to yourself. You shut them out. Besides, people who care about you can probably sense how you feel from the look on your face and your physical demeanour and will be sensitive to your needs.

Accept invitations to social gatherings. Be part of a group. Quite often, the distraction of doing something different that forces you to focus outward rather than inward can help you rise above the pain for a while. You might be surprised to find that you can enjoy yourself and that the pain diminishes.

Taking Control

It may also help your self-esteem if you try to do something physically positive, like exercise, that helps give back some reward. For many years I shied away from exercise because I felt too ill and depressed, listing it in my head as 'one of the things Michele can't do because of this thing'. When the despair about my ballooning body shape became too much, I finally started going to body conditioning and aerobics exercise classes. I instantly found that not only did my pain diminish for those couple of hours, but I felt back in tune with my body and began to see it as a source of strength, and something that needed to be nurtured rather than something that just gave me pain. This new feeling helped my self-esteem immensely. There are countless academic studies which establish that exercise can significantly reduce depression and can increase pain tolerance. Obviously, the sort of the exercise that will suit you will depend on your condition and your lifestyle. Gentle exercise such as walking is an excellent body strengthener and it is worth trying to start a regular regime.

Think Positive

Just thinking positively about your condition can give a boost to your health. Learn to accept what has happened to you and do not let it get in the way – search for other challenges and opportunities rather than obstacles. If you find yourself sinking into a depression about your illness, try to see it not as a sentence, but as a rough patch which you will survive and learn from. Make a conscious effort to find at least one thing to be optimistic about when you are down – a new outfit or holiday or simply the flowers in the garden. Do not bottle up negative emotions as these can easily turn into resentful anger. If you cannot cry or rant, writing down all your feelings (for your eyes only) may help to validate them and help you accept them.

Reducing Anxiety – Finding Support

When will it end? Where can I get help? What is wrong with me? Clinical psychologist Susan Heitler says that the best antidote to anxiety is information. Do not let your doctor fob you off with inadequate explanations of your condition and the treatments available. If this does happen you can keep anxiety at bay by doing your own research. Some hospital departments have specific leaflets about conditions like thrush (yeast infection) and cystitis which can be a good source of information. Find out about the medical libraries in your area; there you can look things up under specific subject areas, and then scour through the latest research. Women's magazines constantly give coverage to new research, so keep an eye out for anything relevant to you.

You could also ring up some of the better ones and ask if the magazine has ever featured an article on your condition. If so, they are usually quite happy to send you a copy. If your doctor does not have the time to talk through your condition and its implications with you, he or she may be able to refer you to some source where you can find the relevant information.

Self-help Groups

Communicating with other women who have the same condition can not only expand your information sources, but can also provide vital support and encouragement. You will be talking with people who *really* understand what you are going through. Contact with other women can either be established in face-to-face group meetings, or in the form of a helpline or newsletter, or, if you are really lucky, all three!

Joining a support network has been the most enormous help. It has put me back in charge of my life and my body – given me back my confidence and eased my fears.
HELEN, 25, TALKING ABOUT THE VESTIBULITIS SUPPORT GROUP
WHICH MEETS ONCE MONTHLY.

The Pelvic Inflammatory Disease Support Network in the UK operates by newsletter which comes out twice a year and many women use this as a forum to tell their stories and share their successes. They find it an invaluable source of information and is it can be sent anywhere, no woman has any reason to feel isolated. As one woman explains in a letter published in 1993:

The newsletter certainly helped me, especially in the early days when I knew nothing about PID and always thought tests showed results. It was through the newsletter that I learnt about hot water bottles – not one doctor or specialist ever mentioned the relief that can bring.

If there is no self-help network in your area, perhaps you could try to set one up. There are many groups and resources available which provide guidance in establishing self-help groups.

Relaxation Techniques

Like many other chronic pain sufferers, I often experience a vicious circle between pain levels and stress. When I am under pressure my vestibulitis seems to be agonizing, and the misery and frustration I then feel makes my physical symptoms even worse. Both pain levels and stress can be dramatically reduced by relaxation and meditation techniques. Joining a yoga, meditation or tai chi class will help you to develop proper skills in this area. Alternatively, there are many organizations producing relaxation and breathing exercise tapes and videos to allow you to practice at home. Recently, creative visualization techniques have become quite popular, especially for chronic illness such as HIV and cancer. Using self-hypnosis and relaxation techniques, you are encouraged to literally visualize the pain disappearing, shrinking it in your mind. Many people say they have found it extremely effective; it is also good to do something for yourself when you feel that everything has been taken out of your hands by healthcare professionals. Here are some general guidelines on relaxation which you might like to try as a starter – perhaps get a friend or partner to read through as you practise.

Make sure that you will be undisturbed for 15 to 20 minutes. Wearing loose clothing, sit either in a comfortable chair or on the floor supported by pillows. Try to empty your mind of distracting thoughts and become aware of your body resting the chair – your muscles, the heaviness of your body and the rhythm of your breathing. Your breathing should be gentle and coming from your stomach rather than your chest. Feel the air passing gently across the back of your throat and each time you breathe out you will feel heavier, calmer and more relaxed.

THE EMOTIONAL EFFECTS OF PAINFUL SEX

Begin by tensing your arms and hands. Make tight fists and hold your hands and arms tight for a few seconds, then gradually relax your fingers and loosen your arms, becoming aware of the relaxed sensation as it spreads from your shoulders to your fingertips.

Take a deep breath then raise your shoulders, pushing them up and back as if doing a giant shrug. Hold it for a moment then relax. Let your shoulders, arms and hands rest and become heavy; feel yourself resting back into the chair.

Taking a deep breath then tense your stomach by making the muscles tight. Hold for a few seconds and relax. Continue by tensing and relaxing your legs and feet, stretching them out in front of you.

Enjoy five or ten minutes at the end relaxing and quietly being aware of your breathing. Imagine yourself somewhere particularly special – on a beach, by a lake or in a beautiful garden. Feel the sensations you would experience if you were really there.

If you practise this at least three times a week you will learn to relax more quickly and deeply when either intense pain or stress strikes. I sometimes combine breathing techniques with auto-suggestion. This involves emptying your mind of distractions and concentrating on your own word or phrase such as 'I will be healthy', or the 'the pain will subside', repeating it either aloud or silently. Another useful technique is autogenic training. Therapists trained in this technique believe that by silently repeating a particular set of phrases, patients can induce various physical sensations. As you relax, you concentrate on the relevant part of your body and repeat in your mind statements like 'I feel warmth flowing through me,' or 'my 'heartbeat is slow and regular'. Complementary therapies can also promote relaxation (*see Chapter 6*).

Chapter 5
INFERTILITY

Women who have experienced some of the conditions mentioned in this book may also be affected by fertility problems. Their conditions may have detrimentally affected their sexual functioning and therefore conception is difficult. Or their conditions may have left them with physical problems which disrupt fertility. Natural fertilization and the maintenance of pregnancy depend on a series of complex and interrelated events. A woman's body must be able to do the following to conceive and carry a carry a baby to term:

- Ovulate regularly.
- Receive sperm into her vagina.
- Maintain adequate female hormone levels in order to produce cervical mucus, aid the implantation of the embryo and maintain the pregnancy.
- Have healthy fallopian tubes to allow the sperm to travel through them.
- Have a healthy uterus to support the implantation of the embryo and foetal growth.

Any defect in these functions will affect a woman's fertility; 'treatment', if it is required, will depend ultimately on the cause of the problem. If not detected and treated early, gonorrhoea, chlamydia and bacterial vaginosis can lead to pelvic inflammatory disease which, if severe, can damage internal reproductive organs, eventually causing infertility. Overall, 30 per cent of infertility is due to pelvic infection. Endometriosis can also affect fertility in a number of ways. The endometrial tissue may interfere with ovulation or implantation of the fertilized ovum. If a woman has undergone a hysterectomy as a form of treatment for endometriosis, then some, or all of her reproductive organs will have been removed, rendering her sterile.

If you have previously suffered any of the above conditions and have been trying to conceive for longer than 12 months without success, then it is important that the actual cause of infertility be investigated as soon as possible. You should not assume automatically that because you have had a 'risk' illness that you are responsible for your lack of conception; your partner should also be investigated. Depending on the cause of infertility, there are a number of possible treatment options open to you. I would like to add that new research is constantly being pursued in this area. The information and statistics below are relevant when going to press, but as these practices are constantly being modified, please check out the best procedures for yourself.

Ovulation Stimulating Drugs

Some women have problems conceiving because they are not ovulating properly. There are a number of reasons for this including premature menopause, ovarian cysts and endometrial implants. If there is a disorder of this nature, the most effective treatment is the administration of ovulation stimulating drugs (fertility drugs). These currently have a very high success rate, but there is a 12 to 15 per cent chance of multiple births. Many women also experience side-effects such as mood swings and nausea from the drugs. Also the sex on demand that this treatment requires can be very demoralizing and hard to maintain.

Oestrogen

In order for sperm to penetrate the cervix and swim upstream into the fallopian tubes, the mucus in the cervix needs to be of a good quality and free from infection. Occasionally the mucus can be of poor quality, or hostile to the man's sperm. Oestrogen can be given prior to ovulation which will stimulate the production of more favourable mucus.

Surgical Treatments

The availability of new and better microsurgical and laser surgery techniques has greatly improved the success rate of gynaecological surgery. Adhesions, blockage and scarring of one or both fallopian tubes due to infections, pelvic inflammatory disease or endometriosis are particularly suited to treatment by this kind of surgery, but ensure that you are treated by a specialist in tubal repair.

Artificial Insemination

This refers to the practice of mechanically introducing into the vagina sperm obtained through masturbation. The sperm donor can be a husband or partner, friend or anonymous donor. This method is useful when the cause of infertility is that the woman does not desire, or cannot have intercourse, or the quality of her partner's sperm is poor. To qualify for this treatment, the woman must have a healthy uterus and one healthy ovary and fallopian tube.

Gamete Intrafallopian Transfer (GIFT)

This involves the transfer of ova and sperm directly into the fallopian tubes where fertilization can take place. In this procedure the woman's eggs are retrieved by laparoscopy after ovulation is induced. A semen sample is collected from the partner, then both egg and sperm are transferred back into the fallopian tube. Following the transfer, the hormone progesterone is administered daily until implantation of the embryo takes place. Treatment of infertility by this technique is used in instances of endometriosis, ovarian failure and tubal adhesions which may be caused by PID. This technique can also be used with donor sperm and donor eggs.

In-vitro Fertilization

This technique bypasses the fallopian tubes completely by fertilizing the egg outside the body in a special laboratory dish. The woman can use her own eggs for this technique, or those from an egg donor, but at the moment demand for egg donors far outweighs supply. In-vitro fertilization (IVF) is mainly performed on women with blocked or damaged fallopian tubes. The woman must have a healthy uterus and at least one normal ovary. IVF can also help when the woman's cervical mucus is 'hostile' to her partner's sperm, because fertilization takes place outside the womb and the fertilized egg is transferred back to the fallopian tubes, bypassing the cervix. The success rate of in-vitro fertilization is not startlingly high; in 1987, 7000 women were treated using IVF with 760 live births resulting.

Other non-medical options that are open to infertile couples who wish to become parents include adoption, fostering and surrogacy, and are all worth considering.

Other Causes and Treatments of Infertility

Infections are not the only conditions that can disrupt fertility. Women with vaginismus may have perfectly healthy vaginas and reproductive organs, but the inability to take any form of penetration means that it is difficult, if not impossible, for them to receive sperm into the vagina. They may be very fearful of giving birth. Male sexual dysfunction such as impotence can be another reason why a couple cannot conceive. Both of these conditions can be overcome with appropriate therapy and counselling.

Women with vulval pain, thrush (yeast infection), cystitis and interstitial cystitis may have similar problems to women with vaginismus. Their ability to receive sperm may be restricted by their frequent inability to have intercourse. These women, together with lesbian women and others who find penile penetration difficult or undesirable may be able to use self-insemination as a means to conceive. This involves inserting a well-lubricated sterile syringe filled with sperm into the vagina yourself, or you can ask a friend or partner to do it for you. With this method there is no potentially painful thrusting involved and you can choose a time when you are most fertile and relatively pain-free, if possible. Your doctor, gynaecologist and numerous women's and lesbian health centres will be able to give you safe instructions on how to do this properly. For women with vulval pain, the fear of giving birth may be overcome by the prospect of the many anaesthetizing drugs now available. Women can have a choice of specific local treatments such as local anaesthetic injections on the vulva, or an epidural, which anaesthetizes the whole area, or a caesarean section birth where the baby is delivered via an incision in the lower abdomen rather than the vagina.

Coping With Infertility

Although society heavily sanctions the view that motherhood is the proper and correct path for women, a paradox remains. When it is difficult for a woman to fulfil her maternal longings, the services available to her are unjustifiably limited. In Britain, the NHS waiting lists for fertility treatments are very long and many people are forced into the private sector to undergo very expensive treatments which may not be successful.

Unfortunately, the emotional significance of infertility, especially for a women whose fertility has been affected by illness, is often played down or ignored within medical fertility services. As a result, these emotional needs are not met. Placing yourself on the treatment merry-go-round can lead to a lot of heartache and confusion , and you may need to ask for counselling and support to help you through it. It is advisable to begin to come to terms with infertility *before* you even start treatment, as this way you can avoid using seeking treatment as a 'denial' of what has happened to your body. It is important to allow yourself to experience grief, as George Christie, an Australian psychotherapist who has studied psychological issues in infertility explains:

> *Just as a couple who have suffered a stillbirth need to mourn their loss before they start another pregnancy, so should a couple mourn the loss of their fertility and their idealized fantasy child before embarking on any alternative route to parenthood.*

He also observes that infertility can be threatening to your sexual identity, making you feel less desirable and capable. The individual or couple has to accept almost a new sexuality, where sexuality and procreation are separated. Other questions you need to consider before looking for treatment include: Am I physically and emotionally prepared for this? Is this what I want, or am I just responding to societal pressures, or pressures from my partner and/or family? Once you have started treatment, ask yourself how much is *too* much. Have I had enough? How many disappointments can I take? How long can I put up with the disruption to my life?

If you choose to, or are forced to give up, this does not mean you are a 'failure'. Realize that you may never have a child, try and accept this – get help if you need it – and then you can try to re-evaluate your goals. There are many specialist counsellors and self-help groups dealing with infertility issues. Accepting that you may be childless may actually signal success and show you how you can come to terms with disappointments in the face of adversity.

Chapter 6

CHOOSING A COMPLEMENTARY THERAPY

As some of the conditions mentioned in the book cannot necessarily be 'cured' by conventional medicine, many women find it helpful to manage their conditions using orthodox medicine combined with complementary health procedures such as homoeopathy and acupuncture. Indeed, an increasing number of women have found complementary medicine to be far more useful to them than other drugs and have adopted it as a preferred method of treatment. Self-help groups for conditions such as PID, endometriosis and vestibulitis often report encouraging success stories from women who have undergone treatment in the complementary health sector. There are an increasing number of women who have been 'cured' of conditions they have suffered for years.

Seeking out complementary health-care can help you feel more in control of your illness and women often say that they do not ever have to deal with the trauma of begging to be believed and are always taken seriously which is not always the case with conventional doctors. All complementary therapies have several principles in common which seem completely logical, but are often lost of in the high-tech maze of conventional medicine.

- The body, mind and spirit are integrated and good health comes from a balance of the three.
- The body has a great capacity to heal itself, and illness happens because of a disruption to that natural balance.
- The environment in which people live, their emotional past and their relationships can all affect health.

Each therapy aims to achieve a balanced state of well-being according to its own theories. With this method patients and practitioners become true partners in care, rather than the more unequal patient and expert alliance. The following is a brief summary of how each method works.

Acupuncture

Traditional acupuncture is based on the principle that health is dependent on the balanced function of the body's motivating energy, known as *Chi*. Chi flows through the body, concentrated in a complex series of channels beneath the skin known as meridians and along these channels lie the points by which the acupuncturist regulates the energy flow and bodily health. According to this theory, we get ill because these energies become imbalanced and therefore the aim of treatment is to restore the harmony of energy in the body.

What Will Happen When I Visit an Acupuncturist?

The practitioners will try to determine the nature of the disharmony in the body by careful questioning. He or she will take a detailed history, including asking questions about responses to climate, taste preferences, feelings and phobias; these can all be useful pointers to the imbalance. The practitioner will also take your pulses to determine where the imbalances are. Acupuncture involves inserting fine needles into specific points on the body so that blocked energy will be released and the body can heal itself.

The needles are so fine that there is little discomfort; they are either withdrawn immediately or left for up to 20 or 30 minutes. Not only does acupuncture aid relaxation and boosts energy levels, it has been found to be effective for chronic pain and conditions, and has no side effects. Acupuncture has also been shown to work well with gynaecological conditions such as PID – you may like to seek out practitioners who specialize in gynaecological problems. The practise of acupressure is similar, but uses finger pressure rather than needles to adjust the energy levels.

Shiatsu

Known as Japanese finger pressure therapy, shiatsu springs from the same ancient oriental principles as acupuncture. It works by stimulating the body's vital energy flow in order to promote good health. Instead of using needles, the practitioner uses thumbs, fingers and elbows to press and stretch the meridian energy lines. This has the effect of stimulating the circulation and the flow of lymphatic fluid, working on the nervous system to release toxins and deep-seated tension. On a more subtle level, shiatsu allows you to relax deeply and get in touch with your body's own healing abilities. Accompanied by deep breathing techniques, a shiatsu massage often leaves a feeling of calmness and well-being.

Homoeopathy

The popularity of this method of healing has increased rapidly over the last 20 years and many people, especially women, swear by homoeopathic remedies, often substituting them for orthodox ones. The principle at work in homoeopathy is completely opposite to that of conventional medicine. Instead of treating an ailment with medication that is an 'antidote' or the complete opposite of the ailment, homoeopathy treats 'like with like'. Take insomnia as an example. Conventionally, it is treated by giving drugs which brings on artificial sleep, even though these drugs could cause side-effects or addiction. Homoeopathic treatment, on the other hand, would mean giving the patient a minute dose of a substance which in large doses causes sleeplessness in a healthy person. Similarly, a nettle rash would be treated with a minute dose of something that would cause a nettle rash.

The remedies work by stimulating the body's own healing powers to deal with the cause of the condition, rather than just the symptoms. The catch is that there are hundreds of remedies and the success of the homoeopathic treatment will depend on matching your symptoms up to the right remedy. The practitioner will ask you detailed questions about the general state of your health, symptoms, the health of your family, feelings and emotions to build up a comprehensive picture of you. This will enable the therapist to make an accurate assessment in the search for a remedy. The remedies are usually small white pills which will have no harmful side-effects, although they might make your symptoms worse before they get better. Unfortunately, the results are not instantaneous and often take between six weeks to three months to work.

Modern homoeopathy is based on the discoveries of the eighteenth-century doctor Samuel Hahnemann. He discovered that the progressive dilution of remedies increases their efficacy, which remains the principle adhered to in today's homoeopathic practice. While a single potency, 1c, represents a dilution of 1 part remedy to 99 parts dilutant, the process can be continued to produce potencies of 10, which is 1 part remedy to 999 of dilutant. Paradoxically, after preparation, homoeopathic remedies bear no chemically detectable trace of the original substance on which it is based. Animal, vegetable and mineral derivatives are all used, as well as drugs such as cocaine, morphine and arsenic, but they are all subjected to the progressive dilution process.

Herbal Treatment

Herbal medicines prepared from the roots, flowers, seeds, stems and leaves of plants have been used by most cultures around the world and there are still many herbalists who use this ancient knowledge to great effect today. Out of the thousands of herbs available to help innumerable conditions, the skill of the herbal practitioner is to find the right herbs for you and your condition and to balance them safely. Again, you will be questioned in-depth about your symptoms and then herbs will be administered to you either in the form of an infusion, decoction, ointment, tincture or compress.

Aromatherapy

Aromatherapy uses essential oils extracted from various parts of aromatic plants and trees to promote physical health and well-being. Unlike herbs, homoeopathy and acupuncture, its effects are usually palliative rather than curative, when it comes to chronic problems, but essential oils can play an important role in helping you cope with your symptoms and improving your state of mind. There are many books available on using essential oils, but keep in mind that they are drugs and as such, must be used carefully. Never use large amounts neat, always mix essential oils with a base oil – the general guideline is 5 drops of essential oil to 10 ml of carrier oil. Essential oils should never be taken internally, nor should they generally be applied to the genitals.

There are four simple ways to reap the benefits of essential oils. The oldest and most obvious method is through massage, which allows the oils to be inhaled and absorbed into the body via the skin. Aromatherapy massage has a relaxing effect on the psyche and a therapeutic effect on the blood circulation and lymph system. You can also inhale essential oils by adding a few drops to your bath, or applying them to poultices or compresses then using on the afflicted area. An aromatherapist will discuss your symptoms with you and will decide on a combination of oils to help you. If your symptoms are getting you down, or are exacerbated by stress, an aromatherapy massage by a qualified therapist is one of the most constructive things you can do to treat yourself and help yourself feel better. He or she can also suggest essential oils to use at home for anything from improving your libido to helping your sleep.

Finding Help

These are just a few of the most popular complementary therapies available and there are many others such as hypnotherapy, naturopathy and reflexology which might be able to help you. As you find your way through the various complementary treatments and seek out the ones that suit you, you can feel a renewed sense of purpose and hope which in itself is emotionally and mentally healing. This is not to say that every complementary practitioner has impeccable motives and credentials, and a magic cure. Complementary medicine is still largely unregulated and therefore finding the right therapy or combination of therapies and the right practitioner to suit you is largely a case of trial and error. Because the majority of practitioners work in private practice this can also prove to be expensive. The following are a few guidelines to help you investigate the options.

To find a practitioner, seek personal recommendations from your doctor, friends or a women's health centre. You can also check with the appropriate self-help group or society for recommendations. All of these sources may be able to tell you of treatments that have helped other people, but also try to remember that because complementary treatments look at the individual rather than the illness, what suits and helps one person may not be right for you. A woman in our vestibulitis group, for example, has become 80 per cent better using herbs and acupuncture. I

CHOOSING A COMPLEMENTARY THERAPY

tried the same route, but could not stand the taste of the herbs so the treatment was unsuccessful for me. If you cannot stand the sight of needles, for example, then acupuncture would not be a good choice for you.

Some practitioners, notably acupuncturists and homoeopaths, may have had conventional medical training and background before taking up complementary disciplines. For a wide variety of reasons, you may feel more comfortable consulting someone with a medical background. Keep this in mind while you search for a treatment.

Ensure that you consult someone with a fully accredited training qualification. This can be done by checking the register of the specific professional body. These professional bodies are often happy to give the details of registered practitioners in your area. Although complementary practitioners are trained to help with all sorts of conditions, some of them do have areas of specialization. Check with the professional association, or the place where you sought the referral to find out if there is a practitioner who specializes in gynaecology or women's health.

In Britain, a limited amount of homoeopathy and acupuncture treatment is available on the NHS. Ask your GP for details. Natural health centres which offer a wide range of complementary health services are opening up all over the place. Many of them have open days where you can meet and discuss your needs with a wide range of specialists before committing yourself to treatments.

An ever-increasing range of books is being published in the area of complementary therapies. If budget is a strong consideration, you might like to try some of the self-help measures that they mention as opposed to seeking a consultation. A book may have an approach or describe a treatment which you feel would suit you very well. Books are a useful tool in finding the right help.

BIBLIOGRAPHY

Introduction
1. Glatt, A. E., Zinner, S. H., McCormack, W. M., 'The Prevalance of Dyspareunia', *Obstetrics Gynaecology*, 75 (1990), pp. 433–6.

Chapter 1
1. *Pharmaceutical Journal*, January 3 (1993).
2. Davidson, F., Oates, J. K., 'The pill does not cause "thrush" (yeast infection)', *British Journal of Obstetric Gynaecology*, 92 (1985), pp. 1265–6.
3. Dennerstein, D. J., 'Depro-provera in the treatment of recurrent vulvo-vaginal candidiasis', *Journal of Reproductive Medicine*, 31 (1986), pp. 801–3.
4. Long Island Jewish Medical Center.
5. Highlights from the Third International Symposium on Vaginitis/Vaginosis, Maderia, Portugal, February 1994.
6. As above.
7. Hay, Dr Philip. St George's Hospital, as reported in the *British Medical Journal*, January 1994.
8. Highlights for the Third International Symposium (as above).

9. Knox, Helen. 'Sexual Health Information booklet', West Lambeth Community Care, (NHS) Trust.
10. Westcott, Patsy. *Pelvic Inflammatory Disease and Chlamydia*, London, Thorsons, 1992.
11. As above.
12. Kilmartin, Angela. *Understanding Cystitis*, Arrow Books, 1989.
13. As reported in *Health & Fitness Magazine*, July 1994.
14. *The Lancet*, 14 January 1989.
16. Welch, Jan. *British Journal of Obstetrics and Gynaecology*, October (1993).

Chapter 2

1. Friedrich, F., 'Vulvar Vestibulitis Syndrome', *Journal of Reproductive Medicine*, Vol. 32, No. 2, February (1987).
2. Solomons, C., Melmed, Clive, Heitler, Susan, 'Calcium Citrate for Vulvar Vestibulitis: A Case Report', *The Journal of Reproductive Medicine*, Vol. 36, 12, December (1991).
3. Goetsch, M., 'Vulvar Vestibulitis: Prevalence and Historic Features in a General Gynecologic Practice Population', *American Journal of Obestetrics and Gynaecology*, Vol. 164, No 6, Part 1, June (1991).
4. Marinoff, S., Turner, M., 'Vulvar Vestibulitis Syndrome', *Dermatologic Clinics*, Vol 10, No 2, April (1992).
5. Hanno, Phillip M., 'Interstitial Cystitis: When Should You Suspect It? What Can You Do About It?', *Emergency Medicine*, June 15 (1989).
6. McCormick, N., Vinson, Robert. *Sexual Difficulties Experienced by Women with Interstatial Cystitis*, The Haworth Press, 1988.
7. Barbach, L. *'The Pause', Positive Approaches to Menopause*, Bantam 1994.
8. *The Perineum in Childbirth*, A Survey Conducted by The National Childbirth Trust 1993.
9. As above.

Chapter 3

1. Berger, Gary S., Westrom, L. V., eds. *Pelvic Inflammatory Disease*, New York, Raven Press, 1992.
2. *Health of the Nation Report*, Department of Health, 1993.
3. Vaginal Douching.
4. Beard, R. W., 'Clinical Features of Women with Chronic Lower Abdominal Pain', *British Journal of Obstetrics and Gynaecology*, Vol. 95, February (1988), pp. 153–61.
5. The Endometriosis Society, UK.
6. *The International Journal of Fertility & Menopausal Studies*, Jan-Feb, 38 (1), (1993), pp. 22–7.
7. *American Journal of Obestrics and Gynaecology*, Feb., 162, (1990), pp. 574–6.
8. Reinisch, June M., Beasley, Ruth. *The Kinsey Institute New Report on Sex*, Penguin, 1990, pp. 446 (same ref for diagram of hysterectomy).
9. 'Sexuality After Hysterectomy', Obstetrics and Gynaecology, 81(3), (1993) March, pp. 357–62.

Chapter 4

1. Heitler, Susan. *The Vulval Pain Newsletter*, Fall (1993).
2. Valins, Linda. *'When a Woman's Body Says No to Sex'*, Penguin 1993.
3. Heitler, Susan, as above.
4. *The G-Spot*.

Appendix 1

USEFUL ADDRESSES

UK

General Medical Information and Counselling for Women's Health Issues

The Medical Advisory Service
10 Barley Mow Passage
London W4 4PH
0181-994 9874

Women's Health
52 Featherstone Street
London EC1Y 8RT

British Pregnancy Advisory Service
7 Belgrave Road
London SW1V 1QB
0171-222 0985

Marie Stopes Family Planning and Health Care
Well Woman Centre
108 Whitfield Street
London W1P 6BE
0171-388 0662

Medway Women's Health Information and Support Service
The White House
Riverside
Chatham
Kent ME4 4SL
01634-407821

Women's Health Advice Centre
1 Council Road
Ashington NE63 8RZ
01670-853977

Women's Health Information and Support Centre
95A Mount Pleasant
Liverpool L3 5TB
0151-707 1826

Midlife Matters
32 Gwynne Road
Parkstone
Poole
Dorset BH12 1AS
01202-735287

British Association for Counselling
1 Regent Place
Rugby
Warwickshire CV21 2PJ
01788-578328

USEFUL ADDRESSES

Support Groups

The Herpes Association
41 North Road,
London N7 9DP
0171–607 9661 (office) 071–609 9061 (helpline)

Interstitial Cystitis Support Group (ICSG)
Council for Voluntary Service
13 Hazelwood Road
Northampton NN1 1LG

The National Childbirth Trust
Alexandra House
Oldham Terrace
Acton
London W3 6NH
0181–992 8637

PID Support Network
c/o Women's Health
52 Featherstone Street
London EC1Y 8RT

Endometriosis Society
35 Belgrave Square
London SW1X 8QB
0171–235 4137

Hysterectomy Support Network
c/o 3 Lynne Close
Green Street Green
Orpington
Kent BR6 6BS

National Association for the Childless
318 Summer Lane
Birmingham B19 3RL
0121-359 4887

Complementary Therapies

Pain Wise UK
33 Kingsdown Park
Tankerton, Kent CT5 2DT
01227-277886

Women's Nutritional Advisory Service
PO Box 268
Lewes
East Sussex BN7 2QN
01273-487366

The Relaxation for Living Trust
168-170 Oatlands Drive
Weybridge
Surrey KT13 9ET

Positive Health Centre
101 Harley Street
London W1
0171-935 1811

British Medical Acupuncture Society
Newton House
Newton Lane
Whitley
Warrington WA4 4JA
01925-730727

USEFUL ADDRESSES

Council for Acupuncture
179 Gloucester Place
London NW1 6DX

Society of Homoeopaths
2 Artizan Road
Northampton NN1 4HU
01604-21400

British Homoeopathic Association
27a Devonshire Street
London W1N 1RJ
0171-935 2163

British Naturopathic and Osteopathic Association
1-4 Suffolk Street
London SW1Y 4HG
0171-930 9254/8

National Institute of Medical Herbalists
9 Palace Gate
Exeter EX1 1JA
01392-426022

Sexual Counselling

Institute of Psychosexual Medicine
11 Chandos Street
Cavendish Square
London W1M 9DE
0171-580 0631

Women's Therapy Centre
6–9 Manor Gardens
London N7 6LA
0171–263 6200

Association of Sexual & Marital Therapists
PO Box 62
Sheffield S10 3TS
0114–2303901

Relate
Contact your telephone directory for your local branch.

USA

General Women's Health Groups and Support Groups

Boston Women's Health Book Collective
240A Elm Street
Somerville
MA 02144
(617) 625 0271

Women's International Network
187 Grant Street
Lexington 02173
Massachusetts
(617) 862 9431

American Social Health Association/HPV
Post Office Box 13827
Research Triangle Park
North Carolina 27709

USEFUL ADDRESSES

The Vulval Pain Foundation
Post Office Drawer 177
Graham
North Carolina 27253
(910) 226 0704/8518

Interstitial Cystitis Association
PO Box 1553
Madison Square Station
New York
NY 10159
(212) 979-6057

Hysterectomy Eductional Resources and Services
HERS Foundation
422 Bryn Mawr Avenue
Bala Cynwyd
Pennsylvannia 19004
(215) 667 7757.

Complementary Therapies

American Association of Naturopathic Physicians
2366 Eastlake Avenue
East Seattle
Washington 98102

Homoeopathic Educational Services
212 Kitteredge Street
Berkeley, CA 94704

National Center for Homoeopathy
801 North Fairfax Street
Suite 306
Alexandria
VA 22134

International Foundation for Homoeopathy
2366 Eastlake Avenue E
No 301
Seattle WA 98102

American Holistic Medical Association
4101 Lake Boone Trail No. 201
Raleigh, NC 27607
(919) 787 0116

Sexual Counselling

Women's Therapy Centre
80 East 11th Street
Suite 101
New York
NY 10003
(212) 420 1974

Marital and Family Therapy
1100 17th Street NW
10th Floor
Washington DC
(202) 452 0109

USEFUL ADDRESSES
Australia

General Women's Health Centres

Women's Information Switchboard
122 Kintone Avenue
Adelaide 5000
(618) 223 1244

Women's Health Care Association
100 Aberdeen Street
Northbridge
Western Australia 6000
(09) 335 8214

Women's Health Resource Collective
653 Nicholson Street
North Carlton
Victoria 3054
(03) 380 9974

Women's Information Services
280 Adelaide Street
Brisbane
Queensland 4000

Women's Service for Health
60 Droop Street
Footscray
Victoria 3011
(03) 689 9588

Women's Health Information Resource Collection
653 Nicholson Street
North Carlton
Victoria 3054
(03) 387 8702/380 9974

Robert Sinclair – Vulval Dermatologist
Silverton Place
101 Wickham Terrace
Brisbane 4000

Endometriosis Association (Victoria)
37 Andrew Cres
Croydon, Victoria
(03) 879 1276

Hysterectomy Support Group (Victoria)
(03) 802 0329

Complementary Therapies

The Wholistic Practitioners Network
1st Floor, 17 Randall Street
Surry Hills
New South Wales 2010
(02) 211 3811

Sexual Counselling

Australian Psychological Society
191 Royal Parade
Parkville
Victoria 3052
(03) 347 2622

USEFUL ADDRESSES

New Zealand

General Women's Health Groups

The Health Alternatives for Women Inc.
PO Box 884
Christchurch
(03) 796 970

Auckland Women's Health Collective
Women's Health Centre
63 Ponsonby Road
Ponsonby
Auckland
(09) 765 173

Auckland Women's Health Council
10 Carlton-Gore Road
Auckland 1

Wellington Woman's Health Collective
10 Kensington Street
PO Box 9172
Wellington
(04) 856 383

The Hutt Valley Endometriosis Support Group
PO Box 31279
Lower Hutt
(04) 661 024

Complementary Health

The Institute of Classical Homoeopathy
PO Box 19–502
Auckland 7

The New Zealand Acupuncture Association
21 Taharoto Road
Takpuna
Auckland

Health Resource Networking Directory
PO Box 7264
Wellesley Street
Auckland 1

Sexual Counselling

Association of Psychotherapists Incorporated New Zealand
40 Goodall Street
Mosgiel
Near Dunedin

Psychological Society of New Zealand
PO Box 4092
Wellington
(04) 899 926

INDEX

abdominal pain 18, 63–6, 80
   chlamydia 18
   interstitial cystitis 42
abnormal tenderness 7
abortion 68
abscesses 70
acupuncture 111–13
   interstitial cystitis 45–6
   pelvic inflammatory disease 72
   allergic reaction 4, 35
anaemia 8, 12
   thrush 8
anal sex 14
anger 84, 86
antibiotics 71
   bacterial vaginosis 17
   chlamydia 19
   cystitis 22
   gonorrhoea 69
   interstitial cystitis 43
   thrush (yeast infection) 9, 11
antidepressants 44
anti–fungal treatments
   thrush (yeast infection) 9
   vulval vestibulitis 35
   vaginal dryness 47
anus 21, 55, 69
   herpes simplex 26
anxiety 47, 81, 86, 92, 100
aromatherapy 115
   childbirth 59
   cystitis 23
   herpes simplex 28
   menopause 51
   thrush (yeast infection) 11
artificial insemination 106

back pain 67, 76
bacteria 16
   cystitis 20–2
   episiotomy 58
   pelvic inflammatory disease 70, 73
bacterial vaginosis 9, 12, 15–17, 61, 105
bartholins glands 35
biopsies 35
bladder
   cystitis 20
   endometriosis 76
   interstitial cystitis 44
   vulval vestibulitis 40
bladder cancer 43
bladder distention 44
bleeding (abnormal)
   chlamydia 18
   endometriosis 76
   menopausal dryness 73

caesarean section 108
cancer 81
candida albicans 8, 11–13
candida galbrata 13
cap (diaphragm)
   chlamydia 20
   cystitis 24, 61
   thrush (yeast infection) 9
cervix 4,5, 19, 26, 61, 63–4, 68–9, 106
cervical erosion 64–5
cervical mucus 104, 107

cervical smear 7, 31, 65, 89
childbirth 55–61, 79
chlamydia 12, 18–20, 61
   pelvic inflammatory disease 68–9, 72, 104
clitoris 3, 32
coil (IUD) 63, 68, 80
complementary therapy 111–18
condoms
   chlamydia 20
   genital warts 30, 61
   thrush (yeast infection) 9, 13
constipation 63
contraceptive sponge 17
cortisone 38, 51
counselling 86, 97
cranberry juice 23–4
cystitis *ix, xv*, 20–25
   persistent cystitis 24–5
   thrush (yeast infection) 14
   vaginal dryness 47–8, 108
cysts 76–8

depression 80, 83, 87, 92
diabetes 12
diagnosis *xvi*, 90
   endometriosis 78
   pelvic inflammatory disease 65
   thrush (yeast infection) 9
   vulval vestibulitis 34
diet

INDEX

interstitial cystitis 45
pelvic inflammatory disease 71
thrush (yeast infection) 11
vulval vestibulitis 40
dihydroergotamine 74
douching 16, 70
dyspareunia *xi*

ectopic pregnancy 65
emotional effects 53, 74, 84, 85–103
endometriosis 17, 64, 70–71, 74–5, 105–6, 11
episiotomy *xiii*, 55–60
evening primrose oil 41
exercise 99

fallopian tubes 4, 19, 68, 71, 76, 81, 104–6
fertility *xiii, xiv*, 66, 77
fertility treatments 109
fingering 73
focal vulvitis 32
foreplay 47, 53, 62, 97

garlic 11
genital warts 29–30
GIFT 110
gonorrhoea 69, 105
guilt 86
GUM clinic 45, 67

herbal treatments 115
cystitis 23
herpes simplex 28
menopause 51
pelvic inflammatory disease 72
thrush (yeast infection) 12
herpes simplex 25–9
HIV *xv*, 87, 102
homoeopathy (treatments) 111–13
childbirth 59
cystitis 22
herpes simplex 27
pelvic inflammatory disease 72
vaginismus 54
hormone balance
endometriosis 76
infertility 104
thrush (yeast infection) 9
vaginal dryness 47–9
vulval vestibulitis 36
hormone treatments 79–80
HPV (human papilloma virus) 29–31
vulval vestibulitis 36
HRT (hormone replacement therapy) 50–1, 74, 80
hypnosis 102
interstitial cystitis 45
vaginismus 54
hysterectomy 75, 81–4

implants 76, 77, 79–80
impotence 96, 108
in vitro fertilisation 107
infection 53
   infertility 104–10
   endometriosis 75
   pelvic inflammatory disease 65–8
   interstitial cystitis 22, 42–7, 108
   vulval vestibulitis 40
internal examination 4–6
internal pain (causes) 63–84
interstitial cystitis 22, 42–7, 108
   vulval vestibulitis 40
isolation *ix*, *xiv*, 86, 92
IUD *see* coil

laporoscopy 63, 66, 71, 74, 107
lesbians 62, 95, 108
libido 47, 93
lichen sclerosis 51–2
live yoghurt
   bacterial vaginosis 17
   thrush (yeast infection) 10
lubrication
   cystitis 24
   dryness 47–50, 81
   emotional problems 92–4
   thrush (yeast infection) 13
   vulval vestibulitis 39–42
masturbation 95–6, 106

menopausal atrophic vaginitis 47–50
menopause
   dryness 47
   endometriosis 79
   lichen sclerosis 52
   hysterectomy 83
menstruation *see* periods
menstrual cycle 78–80
men's symptoms
   chlamydia 18, 68–9
   gonorrhoea 69
   trichomoniasis vaginalis 15
   thrush (yeast infection) 13
   warts 30
miscarriage 17

non–bacterial cystitis 22; *see also* cystitis
non–gonoccal urethritis 19, 68
non–specific urethritis 19, 68

oestrogen
   endometriosis 79–80
   infertility 106
   menopause 48–50
   vulval vestibulitis 39–40
oral contraceptive pill
   cervical erosion 64
   cystitis 24
   endometriosis 79
   progesterone only 10
oral sex 28, 95

INDEX

oral treatments 10
orgasm 49
ovaries 71, 74, 76, 81
ovarian residue 83
ovulation 76, 104
   thrush (yeast infection) 9
ovulation residue 83
ovulation stimulation 105–6
oxalates 37–8

painful sex (incidence of) *xi*
pain management 57, 87, 102
pelvic cavity 76
pelvic congestion 73–5
pelvic examination 89
pelvic inflammatory disease
   xiii, 16–17, 65–73, 105–6, 111
   chlamydia 19
   self–help groups 101
pelvic pain 70, 73, 75, 79
pelvic venography 74
periods (abnormal symptoms)
   chlamydia 18
   endometriosis 75, 77, 79
   pelvic congestion 73
   thrush (yeast infection) 9
perineum 3, 55, 59
Ph balance 70
pregnancy
   bacterial vaginosis 17
   endometriosis 78–9
   fertility 104
   herpes simplex 29

premature labour 16
psychological effects *xii, xiv*
   hysterectomy 83
   infertility 109
   pelvic congestion 73
   vaginismus 52–3
psychotherapy 86, 97

rape *xii*
recurrent thrush (yeast infection) 12–14
reinfection
   herpes simplex 29
   thrush (yeast infection) 13–14
relationships 53, 81, 86, 91
relaxation techniques 102
remedies 114
reproductive organs 63, 105
retrograde menstruation 76
retroverted uterus 64–5, 78

salpingitis 65
salt baths
   thrush (yeast infection) 14
   vulval vestibulitis 41
sanitary towels 58, 62
scar tissue 57, 58, 64
   endometriosis 76
self-esteem 86, 98–9
self-help groups 101, 111, 116
   see appendix
self image 84
sex positions 95, 97

sex therapy 46, 53, 86, 97
sex toys 62, 96
sexuality *xiii, xv, xvi,* 103, 109
   interstitial cystitis 46–7
   hysterectomy 83–5
sexual problems 91–4
sexual satisfaction 95
sexual transmitted disease
    (STD's) 4, 16, 18, 47
shiatsu 113
Skene's glands 35
stitches 57, 60
stigma *xiv*
stress 47
surgery 64, 72, 10
swabs (vaginal) 7, 9, 70

TENS pain relief 44
thrush (yeast infection) *ix, xiv, xv,* 7–14, 61, 71–2, 108
   bacterial vaginosis 16
   chronic thrush 13–14
   cystitis 14–15
   dryness 47
   vaginismus 53
   vulval vestibulitis 33–5
treatments for conditions 4
   bacterial vaginosis 17
   cervical erosion 65
   childbirth problems
   chlamydia 19–20
   cystitis 22–5
   endometriosis 78–80
   herpes simplex 27

menopause 50
pelvic inflammatory disease 71
pelvic congestion 74
thrush (yeast infection) 9
trichomoniasis vaginalis 14–15
vaginismus 53
vulval vestibulitis 38–42

ultrasound test 70, 74
unprotected sex 19
urethra 3, 32, 42,
   cystitis 20–21, 26
   gonorrhoea 69
   menopause 48
urinary frequency 20–21, 42–5
urinary pain 18–19, 20–21, 42–5, 76
urinary tract infections; *see* cystitis 20–22
urine tests 19, 21
uterine cancer 83
uterus 4, 63, 71, 76, 78, 81, 104, 107

vagina 2–3
   arousal 64
   cystitis 20
   vaginismus 54
   vulval vestibulitis 33
vaginal discharge
   bacterial vaginosis 16
   cervicitis 19

INDEX

chlamydia 18
thrush (yeast infection) 8
vaginal dryness 32, 47–50 *see* menopausal atrophic vaginitis
vaginal examinations 54–5
vaginal infections/irritations 1–31
vaginal itching 51
   bacterial vaginosis 16
   dryness 47
   herpes simplex 26
   thrush (yeast infection) 8
   vulval vestibulitis 32–4
   vulvodynia 36
vaginal muscles 52–5
vaginal pain 32–62
vaginal rings 50
vaginal swabs *see* swabs
vaginismus 5, 52–5, 89–90, 108
vestibule 3, 33, 39

vulva 2–3, 30
vulval cancer 31, 52
vulval pain 32–62, 108
   bacterial vaginosis 16
   dryness 47
   genital warts 30
   herpes simplex 26
   interstitial cystitis 42
   lichen sclerosis 51
   trichomoniasis vaginalis 14
vulval vestibulitis *x*, *xiv*, 5, 12, 32–42
   vaginismus 53
   self help 101, 111
Vulvar Pain Foundation 37; *see* appendix
vulvodynia 36

yeast infection *see* thrush
young women
   chlamydia 18

Of further interest

CYSTITIS

How to prevent infection and inflammation

Angela Kilmartin

Cystitis, with or without bacteria, causes pain, burning, frequency and sometimes backache and fever. It has plagued women since time began. This book will teach you how to prevent cystitis from even starting and offers plans that can free you from it for good.

Angela Kilmartin, herself a former sufferer, has spent years perfecting a simple and 100-per-cent successful method for preventing bacterial cystitis without the need to take antibiotics or undergo surgery. By taking a careful look at what causes both bacterial and non-bacterial cystitis, this pioneering author gives you the information you need to discover how your cystitis started and what to do to eradicate it

PAIN-FREE PERIODS

Natural ways to overcome menstrual problems
Stella Weller

'It's just something women have to put up with'
'It'll be better once you get older'
'Having a baby ususally helps...'

If you are one of the millions of women who suffer from dysmenorrhoea, or painful periods, advice like the above is not very helpful. You may feel that the only answer is to continue to grin and bear it each month.

But there are many ways you yourself can help to lessen the misery. Stella Weller provides gentle, natural treatments that can be amazingly effective. Dietary advice, yoga, exercise, herbal remedies and other techniques can be combined to provide real relief for period pain, PMS, and other problems associated with menstruation.

OSTEOPOROSIS

The brittle bones epidemic and how you can avoid it

Kathleen Mayes

Thinning, brittle bones, wrist and hip fractures, round-shouldered, stooped senior citizens, loss of height as you grow older...sound familiar? Osteoporosis is on the increase: indeed, it has reached almost epidemic proportions, particularly among postmenopausal women. Treating osteoporosis-related injuries costs millions each year.

The good news is that in many cases, osteoporosis is preventable, and there is much you can do yourself to stop or at least slow down its development. The key is understanding what it is, knowing whether you may be at risk, and being aware of how you can lessen its effects.

This book presents you with a complete overview of the causes and effects of osteoporosis. If you are at risk from osteoprorosis, you owe it to yourself to make the simple changes in your lifestyle which this book suggests. Find out how you too can protect your bones for life.

CYSTITIS	0 7225 2996 1	£4.99
PAIN-FREE PERIODS	0 7225 2856 6	£4.99
OSTEOPOROSIS	0 7225 2509 5	£4.99

All these books are available from your local bookseller or can beordered direct from the publishers.

To order direct just tick the titles you want and fill in the form below:

Name: ....
Address: ....
....
.... Postcode ....

Send to Thorsons Mail Order, Dept 3, HarperCollins*Publishers*, Westerhill Road, Bishopbriggs, Glasgow G64 2QT.

Please enclose a cheque or postal order or your authority to debit your Visa/Access account —

Credit card no: ....
Expity date: ....
Signature: ....

— up to the value of the cover price plus:
UK & BFPO: Add £1.00 for the first book and 25p for each additional book ordered.
Overseas orders including Eire: Please add £2.95 service charge. Books will be sent by surface mail but quotes for airmail dispatches will be given on request.

24-HOUR TELEPHONE ORDERING SERVICE FOR ACCESS/VISA CARDHOLDERS — TEL: 0141 772 2281.